Ethics, Jurisprudence, and Practice Management in Dental Hygiene

VICKIE J. KIMBROUGH, RDH, MBA

CHARLA J. LAUTAR, RDH, PHD

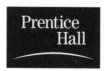

Prentice Hall

Upper Saddle River, New Jersey 07458

Library of Congress Cataloging-in-Publication Data

Kimbrough, Vickie.
  Ethics and practice management in dental hygiene / Vickie Kimbrough, Charla Lautar.
     p. cm.
  Includes bibliographical references and index.
  ISBN 0-13-019138-8
  1. Dental hygiene—Moral and ethical aspects.   2. Dental hygienists.   3. Dental ethics.
I. Lautar, Charla J.   II. Title.
  [DNLM: 1. Practice Management, Dental—organization & administration. 2. Dental
Hygienists. 3. Ethics, Dental. 4. Legislation, Dental.   WU 77 K49e 2002]
  RK60.5.K563   2002
  174'.96176—dc21

                                                                      2001052368

Publisher: *Julie Levin Alexander*
Senior Acquisitions Editor: *Mark Cohen*
Assistant Editor: *Melissa Kerian*
Editorial Assistant: *Mary Ellen Ruitenberg*
Director of Production and manufacturing: *Bruce Johnson*
Managing Editor for Production: *Patrick Walsh*
Production Liaison: *Alexander Ivchenko*
Manufacturing Manager: *Ilene Sanford*
Manufacturing Buyer: *Pat Brown*
Creative Director: *Cheryl Asherman*
Cover Design Coordinator: *Maria Guglielmo-Walsh*
Formatting: *Pine Tree Composition*
Marketing Manager: *David Hough*
Product Information Manager: *Rachele Triano*
Printer/Binder: *Von Hoffman Owensville*
Copy Editor:
Proofreader:
Cover Design:
Cover Printer: *Phoenix Color*

Pearson Education LTD.
Pearson Education Australia Pty, Limited
Pearson Education Singapore, Pte. Ltd.
Pearson Education North Asia Ltd
Pearson Education Canada, Ltd
Pearson Educación de Mexico, S.A. de C.V.
Pearson Education—Japan
Pearson Education Malaysia, Pte. Ltd
Pearson Education, Upper Saddle River, New Jersey

Notice: The author[s] and the publisher of this volume have taken care that the information and technical recommendations contained herein are based on research and expert consultation, and are accurate and compatible with the standards generally accepted at the time of publication. Nevertheless, as new information becomes available, changes in clinical and technical practices become necessary. The reader is advised to carefully consult manufacturers' instructions and information material for all supplies and equipment before use, and to consult with a healthcare professional as necessary. This advice is especially important when using new supplies or equipment for clinical purposes. The author[s] and publisher disclaim all responsibility for any liability, loss, injury, or damage incurred as a consequence, directly or indirectly, of the use and application of any of the contents of this volume.

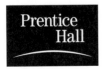

10 9 8 7 6 5 4 3 2 1
ISBN 0-13-019138-8

Contents

CHAPTER 7   ASPECTS OF PRACTICE MANAGEMENT   111

Preface

The information and examples in this book are designed to orient dental hygiene students to clinical practice and its many applications in an office setting. Although dentists, dental practices, and dental hygiene can be generalized, each practice will be unique in its daily operations and policies.

As you read and participate in the exercises, keep in mind that experiences will be unique. In this new millennium, the art and science of dental hygiene continues to progress and evolve. More states have entered into independent or alternative practice settings for experienced dental hygienists.

Upon becoming a registered or licensed dental hygienist, you are encouraged to actively participate in furthering the development of patient education and dental hygiene research as well as your own education. Reach out to communities that are not able to access dental care in a traditional setting and continually stay abreast of the link between periodontal disease and total body health, as patients see the dental hygienist as the oral health care specialist. The knowledge and relationships that build from networking with other professionals will be invaluable.

We hope that you find personal and professional satisfaction in your dental hygiene career and as a member of the dental hygiene profession.

Thank you to the reviewers of this manuscript: W. Gail Barnes, RDH, Ph.D., Assistant Professor, East Tennessee State University; Chris French Beatty, RDH, Ph.D., Associate Professor, Department Chair Texas Woman's University; Barbara Paige, RDH, MS, Ed.D., Professor, Cabrillo College; Angelina E. Riccelli, RDH, MS, Associate Professor and Director, University of Pittsburgh; Donna J. Stach, RDH, M.Ed., Associate Professor, University of Colorado.

ACKNOWLEDGMENTS

Thank you to Dr. Mohamed Elsamahi for useful remarks and suggestions throughout the writing of this text, and to Debi Gerger, RDH, BS, MPH, for her input and case scenarios.

Charla J. Lautar, RDH, PhD

To my sons, Kris, Lenny, and Rik—thank you for your support over the years as I achieved my goals for higher education. And of course, thank you to my mom, Joanne, for her continuous pride in my achievements.

Special thanks to Lori Gagliardi, RDH., MEd, in encouraging me to go forward with this project. I would like to thank the many educators I have been in contact with during my education and those who inspired me as I became involved in dental hygiene education. Special thanks to Dr. Stacy Eastman for being such a great friend and allowing me to bring real life situations into my classroom.

Thank you to my students and faculty members for providing valuable information and feedback even after graduation and participating in this project. Keep in touch and continue to contribute your experiences.

Thank you Debi Gerger, RDH, BS, MPH, for being open and willing to contribute to this project. The gesture is indicative of all educators seeking the highest quality in dental hygiene education.

And of course, to all my friends at table one, your friendship is priceless.

Vickie J. Kimbrough, RDH, MBA

Introduction

The purpose of this book is to help prepare the dental hygienist for dealing with moral, legal, and administrative challenges. It will be of significant help for prospective dental hygienists to have a preview of the nonclinical decisions that they will eventually need to make during their professional careers. Like other health care professionals, dental hygienists will face ethical, legal, and administrative issues that require theoretical preparation. This book is a useful tool in that respect.

Principles exist that guide the relation between dental hygienists and their patients, the moral standards that the public expects from health care providers, patients' entitlements and rights, and the duties of the hygienist towards society. The connection between professional ethics and jurisprudence is intimate. Ethics determines the norms that members of the profession should follow. Jurisprudence and legal guidelines ensure the adherence to such norms. Consequently, discussing the ethical principles that dental hygiene has adopted invites a discussion of the regulations that govern practicing dental hygienists.

Dental hygienists are licensed health care professionals. As members of a profession, they possess attributes that dictate both ethical and legal behavior. Dental hygienists are accountable for their actions, they are required to maintain continuing education, they practice according to a code of ethics developed by a professional association, they perform functions regulated by state practice acts through legislative bodies, and they have their own discipline of knowledge published in professional journals. Therefore, it is logical that a textbook for practice management would also include guidelines for ethical and legal conduct.

An introduction to moral philosophy and moral reasoning provides a background for the study of ethical theories and core values fundamental to a code of ethics. Faced with ethical dilemmas regarding patient care, the dental hygienist is able to use the Code of Ethics developed by the American Dental Hygienists' Association as a guide for decisions pertaining to the practice of dental hygiene. At times, the philosophy of the dental office or the employer's wishes are in conflict not only with the ethics of the individual dental hygienist, but also with the regulation of dental hygiene. Thus, decision-making regarding patient care mandates a consideration of ethics, jurisprudence, and social issues relevant to health care in society. In addition, the dental hygienist needs to be aware of governmental policies and employment regulations that impact the delivery of oral health care in private and public workplace settings.

Upon graduating from dental hygiene school, administrative issues and tasks performed in the dental office on a daily basis may be unfamiliar. Management styles of the dentist and office manager will range from practice to practice. Each office will require the dental hygienist to "fit in" with the style and personality of its practice. It is in the best interest of the dental hygienist to have an adequate understanding of what practice management may entail as related to dental hygiene care.

The practice management information this book covers includes management styles, working as a team member, and the qualities and skills prospective employers look for in a licensed dental professional. Additionally, new technology and computerization have become an integral aspect of providing dental hygiene services. It is now imperative for the dental hygienist to be aware of and learn how to use new technologies. Marketing and public relations may not seem to apply to dental hygiene care; however, interpersonal skills are part of the professional's image and influence how well an individual can market his or her dental hygiene knowledge and clinical expertise. Additionally, dental hygienists want to provide accurate information on restorative materials, as the practice must have patients for both restorative procedures and dental hygiene therapy.

Dental care is health care. However, the dental practice is also seen as a business. If the dental practice is to remain viable and continue delivering oral health care, it must succeed as a business. The practice must charge a fee for its services and handle all the necessary paperwork for billing insurance claims and collecting money. Insuring quality oral health care for all patients in the practice means that scheduling procedures must be designed efficiently, and today's dental hygienist is finding that he or she is responsible for more than continuing care appointments. In addition, more states have begun to allow independent or alternative practice for experienced dental hygienists who have attained additional education. With this, the dental hygienist must become knowledgeable in all aspects of the business of oral health care delivery.

The last five years have brought numerous new technologies to delivering dental and dental hygiene care. Automated probing systems, digital radiography, and computer terminals in each operatory are not a futuristic dream anymore; they are a reality. It is imperative for the dental hygienist to have experience in these treatment modalities. Currently, most dental professionals must learn these advanced skills while they are on the job or during continuing education courses. Additionally, time management for the new graduate continues to be one of the most difficult obstacles to overcome. Becoming familiar with working techniques that assist in time management will be an advantage during the first few months of this new career.

Finally, there are several ways to be compensated as a dental hygienist. For example, benefits can be increased that a career in dental hygiene is a viable source of income, stability, and retirement. Having firsthand knowledge of what benefits are available, or at least negotiable, will increase chances for career longevity. Becoming a dental hygienist can be rewarding in many ways. By understanding dental hygiene as a business, the practice of dental hygiene will be an ensured success.

The practice management portion of this book is designed for dental hygiene students who are about to graduate. This information will assist in familiarizing the new graduate with the many facets of the business that brings oral health care to the public. Some topics discussed throughout the book link ethics with practice management, as the practice of dental hygiene requires knowledge of ethical benefits and consequences. It is hoped that the student will integrate and build on concepts, as new content is presented in each chapter. We have attempted to ensure the uniformity of content throughout the book and to stress the inherent connections between the ethical and practical aspects of the dental hygiene profession. To facilitate learning, there are review summaries, self-test items, individual and group activities, questions for discussion, and case scenarios at the end of each chapter. We hope this book serves as preparation for meeting the challenges of private practice and insures success for the new dental hygienist.

1

Introduction to Moral Philosophy and Moral Reasoning

OBJECTIVES

Upon reading the material in this chapter, you will be able to

1. Define the term *ethics.*
2. Define the terms *deontology* (deontological approach) and *teleology* (telelogical approach).
3. Distinguish between the *utilitarianism* ethical theory and *Kant's* ethical theory.
4. Compare *rule* utilitarianism with *act* utilitarianism.
5. Contrast a *right* with a *duty* and a *right* with a *privilege.*
6. Discuss the role of *social justice* in determining ethical behavior.

INTRODUCTION

The discipline of **ethics** consists of thoughts and ideas about morality. Ethics (or moral thinking) is concerned with studying human behavior, particularly towards other human beings, and the principles that can regulate it. Most ethical thinkers are philosophers, and philosophy differs from social sciences in its tendency to suggest or recommend standards, or norms, of behavior. For example, a sociologist may study the phenomenon of aggression, focusing on the causes of aggression and how some members of society become aggressive under certain circumstances. Similarly, a psychologist may explain why some people fail to develop normal empathic attitudes to others and become indifferent and insensitive to human suffering. A philosopher, on the other hand, would deal with aggression and insensitivity to suffering as violations of several moral values and would propose arguments to support the importance of peaceful and mutually respectful attitudes for human life.

The difference is that science, whether social or physical, is mainly descriptive, while moral philosophy is mainly **normative.** Science analyzes phenomena at depth and explains them. It may also predict future events on the basis of present observations. But ethical philosophy goes beyond studying phenomena at a descriptive level and proceeds to recommend desirable attitudes. Because desirable attitudes are commonly called *norms* ethical thinking that purports to guide human behavior is called *normative ethics.*

Traditionally, the ethical studies that explore the nature of moral judgments and the structure of moral concepts is called *metaethics.* Metaethical studies investigate, for example, the meaning or the significance of what is right or wrong (good or evil) and whether moral judgments are objective or subjective (Honderich, 1995, p. 555). Normative ethics is the branch of metaethics that is concerned with moral recommendations about which acts are right and which are wrong.

The study of normative ethics that is relevant to health care ethics can be divided into two major groups of theories. The first is **deontology.** Advocates of deontological ethics emphasize duties. For them, performing moral duties is not a matter of deliberation or negotiation. A **duty** is an obligation, an act that has to be done or ought to be done regardless of its consequences. In that way, deontological ethics shares with religions the concept of absolute obligation. A deontologist, for example, would expect people to tell the truth, no matter what happens as a result. This is similar to the attitude of a religious person who never lies because it is against the Ten Commandments. Ethical duties are derived from ethical principles and concepts. Some of these duties (e.g., truthfulness) are adopted by health care professions and stated in codes of professional ethics. Other duties (e.g., respect for private property) are incorporated into the legal system, while others (e.g., respect for privacy and helping the poor or elderly) are incorporated into social traditions and customs (Weinstein, 1993, p. 84). Purtilo (1999) defines three basic duties: absolute, prima facie, and conditional (p. 60). An absolute duty is binding under all circumstances. For example, the duty not to kill an innocent person is absolute because we know of no situation in which such killing would be permissible.

Prima facie duties differ in that they are determined by the present situation. The term **prima facie** means *at first glance*, and a prima facie duty is a duty that is made obvious by the circumstances surrounding it. In dentistry, a scenario to illustrate this is treating the patient who is in pain before treating the patient who has come for a routine scheduled appointment. Treating the patient in pain seems to be the right decision even though it may upset the scheduled patient because of unexpected waiting.

A conditional duty is a commitment that comes into being after certain conditions are met. For instance, our society has a duty to support unemployed persons only after they try to learn new skills that may enable them to find jobs or after it becomes obvious that they have no chance to find employment. Similarly, we have a duty to support medical research only after ensuring that it is well designed, feasible, and is concerned with major health problems rather than with academic curiosities. Duties are further discussed in this chapter and in Chapter 2, "Ethical Principals and Core Values."

Thus far, we have discussed the deontological group of theories. Let us examine the second group of theories, which is called *teleological* theories. The term **teleology** is derived from the Greek word for end, or goal. A teleologist will consider the consequences of telling the truth versus the consequences of lying, and may find that lying is morally justified in a specific circumstance. This position, which is also called *consequentialism*, is based on the notion that what matters for morality is the result, or consequence, of an action. Telling a "little white lie" that will do more good than telling the truth counts, for teleologists, as a good action. For instance, a teleologist would say that lying to a known killer about the hiding place of his potential victim is morally good. So the difference between deontologists and teleologists is that the former are concerned with the principle behind an action while the latter are concerned with the results of an action.

ETHICAL THEORIES: A SURVEY OF MORAL THEORIES

Utilitarianism

The first utilitarians were the British philosophers Jeremy Bentham and John Stuart Mill, who lived in the nineteenth century. They argued that the aim of morality is attaining the greatest amount of utility for human beings and identified utility (or usefulness) with happiness. Their theory, which became popular during much of the twentieth century in Britain and North America, is a **consequentialist theory.** Consequentialist (teleological) theories are based in the results of actions rather than in the nature of actions. For instance, if telling a lie can lead to saving an innocent life in a particular situation, it is morally good to tell a lie in that situation. That is, an action is morally right if it leads to desirable results, and is wrong if it leads to undesirable results. Utilitarianism defines the "good consequence," or "desirable result," as the *maximal happiness* in the world (i.e., happiness for most people). According to utilitarianism, suffering is the ultimate evil and happiness is the ultimate good, and the role of morality is to guide us to eliminate suffering and maximize happiness.

Utilitarianism does not recommend that every person pursue only what promotes his or her happiness. Instead, it recommends that all persons act in a way that leads to the least misery and the most happiness (including personal happiness) in the world. The utility principle recommends that we seek the "general" or "total" happiness in society rather than our own personal happiness. However, utilitarians do not ask us to ignore our own happiness, but to view it as a part of total happiness. In that respect, utilitarianism adopts the principle of beneficence, which is discussed in the next chapter. The beneficence principle requires one to do what is good for others without expecting a reward for doing so.

To understand utilitarianism, consider this example. A healthy man knows that his neighbor's daughter needs a kidney transplant to survive after a disease destroyed both her kidneys. He volunteers to have his tissues tested for compatibility with the girl's tissues, and the result turns out to be positive. If he donates his kidney to save the girl's life, he exposes himself to a major surgical operation. He also knows that if he lives with only one kidney, there is a small chance of having a disease in that kidney in the future that may be severe enough to kill him. Donating his kidney would cost him at least some peace of mind. Should he accept this price (i.e., some anxiety about future health) and give the girl one of his kidneys? Utilitarians would encourage him to do so, as long as he is unlikely to be significantly harmed. By saving her life, he makes her and her family and friends happy. He also makes people who advocate benevolent actions happy by giving a good example of benevolent behavior that may inspire others. The outcome of his action, then, would be more happiness in the world, and this agrees with the utility principle.

But utilitarians would not encourage a person who is likely to be harmed by a surgical operation to donate his kidney. As soon as the girl and her family realize that the benevolent man has exposed himself to a great danger they would feel sorry rather than happy and thankful. At the same time, the man's own family and friends would be unhappy if he is harmed. In the end, his action would not add to the total happiness in the world, and is therefore unethical on utilitarian grounds. So utilitarianism does not expect from any individual sacrifices that would not maximize happiness and minimize suffering for the greatest number of people.

When utilitarians discuss happiness, they do not mean any form of happiness. Happiness can be shallow, short-lasting, significant, long-lasting, hedonic (in the form of pleasurable feeling), or intellectual (for example, enjoying an artwork). Short-term happiness is not the aim of utilitarianism. No utilitarian, for example, would encourage a student fond of sports to abandon school to satisfy the passion for sports, or an art lover with limited resources to spend most of an income on collecting paintings. It is also important to recognize that utilitarianism does not construe happiness merely as pleasure. Satisfaction in general, whether it derives from meeting one's basic needs, reading interesting novels, or helping the poor would count as happiness for utilitarians. Another important point is that utilitarians regard reducing suffering (or decreasing unhappiness) equivalent to increasing happiness in the world. A dental hygienist who donates time to a public-aid clinic, thinking that the consequences will bring happiness to others, is guided by the utility principle. If the dental hygienist who donates time to the public-aid clinic instead of working for a salary is not able to provide for his or her children, then this is not following utilitarian principle.

There are two versions of utilitarianism: act utilitarianism and rule utilitarianism. An **act utilitarian** is concerned with individual acts. This person would assert that acting in a certain way (for example, keeping promises) promotes general happiness, and for that reason, it is a good action. A **rule utilitarian,** on the other hand, is more concerned with the rule from which an action is derived. He or she would assert that the goodness of an action depends on whether it is justified by a rule that, if followed, can maximize happiness in the world. There seems to be no substantial difference between the two positions. However, in some situations rule utilitarianism can avoid problems that act utilitarianism cannot. As dental hygienists, we know that polishing teeth can damage tooth structure. Many patients feel that they have not received complete treatment unless the teeth are polished, even though they are told about the disadvantages of polishing and they do not have stains. In order to provide happiness to the patient, the dental hygienist gives the illusion of polishing by sweeping the rubber cup over the surfaces of the teeth with minimal or no pressure. The patient feels the act of polishing and tastes the polishing agent. It is difficult to describe a deceptive act as morally good, yet a rule utilitarian would not agree that the dental hygienist's action was good because adopting the rule that deceiving people in order to please them would not maximize happiness. Rational people would feel unhappy and even angry if they knew that they were deceived in order to be pleased. It would be wrong to suggest to a patient that a procedure was done when in fact it was not.

Is utilitarianism relevant to health care ethics? Yes, because this theory is concerned with reducing suffering, which is one of the main duties of health care providers. Moreover, utilitarianism contributes significantly to the discussion of the problem of fair distribution of health care resources.

The Kantian Ethics

According to Immanuel Kant, the eighteenth century German philosopher, certain acts are morally right because they are intrinsically right, regardless of their consequences or results. Consequences, he asserts, should not matter when the moral value of an action is assessed. Kant even argues that consequences are relevant to practical matters, not to ethics. In the practical realm, one has to ask whether or not an action can lead to good results and act accordingly. For example, a student may decide to study engineering because engineers have good careers. Such a decision is based on consequential (teleological) considerations: Studying engineering qualifies one to enter a stable and rewarding career. When that student decided to be an engineer to enjoy the benefits that result from this decision, he or she was making a consequentialist but purely practical decision. But the situation is different in the moral realm.

In the moral field, there are acts that must be done whether they lead to desirable or undesirable results. Therefore, these acts are moral duties, Kant asserts. These acts lose moral worth when they are done to attain an aim. For example, if you do not tell lies because you want to impress people and get their support or votes, you are either acting practically (from practical motives) or immorally (by trying to exploit ethical principles for material gain). However, if you do not tell lies because you believe that lying is morally wrong, you are acting morally. In other words, you are performing a moral duty. Because Kant's ethics is concerned with duties and reduces moral principles to duties, it was called *deontological* (from the Greek *deon*, meaning obligation).

Kant opposed deriving moral principles from accidental events and contingencies because that could lead to formulating contradictory principles. Suppose that a freedom fighter in Poland during World War II gave the Nazi officers who were interrogating him false information about the identities of his partners. By doing that, he saved their lives and served a good cause. But can we derive from that circumstance a principle that justifies telling lies when it is convenient to do so? Kant's answer is an unequivocal no. For him, ethical principles cannot be a subject for negotiation, nor should they be modified to adapt to new situations when it appears useful to modify them. It is wrong, he believes, to modify one's commitment to truth telling in light of the present circumstances. Moral principles, Kant insists, should be based on solid foundations, then followed with total disregard for the context. If we believe that truth telling is good, we must always tell the truth, even if that leads to great harm in a particular context. Thus, the Polish freedom fighter did not act according to sound moral principles when he lied to the Nazis, in Kant's opinion.

Kant acknowledged that it is sometimes harmful to follow moral principles faithfully. He knew very well that, at least in exceptional cases, we might do better by violating moral principles. But he argued that repeated violations could send a harmful message to people. Violations (or variations) may suggest that one is encouraged to violate moral principles when it seems useful to do so. This seemed alarming to Kant. He believed that interpreting moral principles in a relative way, which permits us to lie today then tell the truth tomorrow, will open the door for moral confusion and chaos. Consequently, moral principles should be absolute (unmodifiable). So the main issue in Kantian ethics is that there are *categorical* (absolute) imperatives (duties) that are inescapable. They can be inferred by reason and should be generalized.

Kant's contention that duties are categorical is very disputable. However, his view that we must treat all persons as ends in themselves, not as means, is widely respected. How does he argue for that principle? According to Kant, every human being is a rational person. Naturally, rational persons appreciate and value their rationality. As a result, they would not accept being used or treated as a means. Their self-respect and respect for the value of rationality would not allow that. It follows that no person should accept being treated as a means to other ends and that every person ought to be treated as an end in herself or himself. This principle is highly esteemed in ethics, and in health care ethics in particular. As will be seen later, it follows from this principle that people should not be treated as objects, and as a result, their well being (and health) should not be treated as a commodity. Using the previous example, the dental hygienist who donates time to a public-aid clinic because it is a *moral* duty— even if this means losing salary, sacrificing leisure time, or denying his or her children small pleasures—to help the disadvantaged, is guided by deontological or Kantian principle.

Virtue Ethics

Virtue ethics places emphasis on character traits of individuals and was advocated by the early philosophers such as Socrates, Plato, and Aristotle. According to them, virtue is the basis of morality. They regarded persons of excellent character as moral persons. That is, a virtuous person is essentially a person who acts morally. The virtue approach to ethics demands that every person think and act in the best way possible for a given situation (Ozar, 1994, p. 4). For example, a virtuous person would advocate fairness and equal respect for people's interests when a conflict between individuals arises and requires mediation or arbitration. He or she would also recommend kindness to animals, honesty in financial dealings, and truth telling. In other words, virtuous people are disposed to think and act morally. This disposition (or readiness to act in certain way) is taken by the proponents of virtue ethics as the guide to moral judgments.

Advocates of virtue ethics expect and require every person to act like a virtuous person. By doing so, they act in a morally good way. This shows that virtue ethics relies on the moral inclination of people with excellent personal qualities to identify the morally right and wrong. Obviously, this approach differs from other systems of metaethics (e.g., deontology and teleology), which rely on rules, principles, consequences, or goals. That is, virtue ethics tells us to act the way a virtuous person would act in a similar situation, while other systems tell us to act according to the principle or rule that suits the situation. Such a principle or rule may derive from Kantian or utilitarian theories, for example.

Historically, the ancient virtue ethics emphasized the cardinal virtues of temperance, justice, courage, and wisdom. In the Middle Ages, Christianity added the theological virtues of faith, hope, and charity. Many feel that a person cannot possess one virtue without the other and that all virtues are interrelated or interdependent. In other words, a person who is courageous and truthful would also be fair and benevolent. But virtue ethics, which was ignored in modern times, is no longer dead. There are contemporary philosophers who think that a focus on virtue, not on abstract principles, can form the basis for morality (Honderich, 1995, p. 901).

SOCIAL PHILOSOPHY

Social philosophy deals with issues like justice, rights, and equality. Problems in medical ethics that belong to the area of social philosophy include, among other things, equal access to health care resources and patients' rights.

Utilitarianism and Justice

Utilitarianism is meant to be a social philosophy as well as a general theory of normative ethics. The utilitarian view of justice is probably the most important component in the social aspect of utilitarianism. Utilitarians understand social justice as a means to happiness. They argue that satisfying basic needs leads to more happiness than does enjoying luxuries. For sure, a nice weekend in Hawaii would make any person feel happy. But there are degrees of happiness. Compare the happiness that a vacationing person in Hawaii would experience with the happiness that a starving, chilled person would experience when fed and warmed. Apparently, the utilitarians are warranted in asserting that satisfying essential needs creates greater pleasure than satisfying less basic needs. Moreover, lacking basic needs, such as adequate food and shelter, is apt to create suffering, while giving up some luxuries is unlikely to produce significant suffering.

Consequently, taking some resources from people who have already satisfied all their basic needs and giving them to those whose basic needs are not satisfied would increase the amount of total happiness in the world. And this is the declared aim of utilitarianism. So justice, as conceived by utilitarians, is a process that is meant to maximize happiness and reduce suffering. It is not an end in itself, though.

The implications of this view of social justice for health care ethics are obvious. A society in which the majority of people are unable to obtain health care cannot be called a happy society. Sickness produces suffering and undermines happiness; and whenever the number of sick or improperly treated people in a society is large, happiness in this society is limited. It follows then that making health care resources available for all or most members of society is essential for keeping the level of happiness in that society sufficiently high. This is how utilitarians justify the necessity of distributing health care resources (or goods) fairly among all people. It is important, however, to notice that utilitariansim does not call for complete equality, but for the extent of equality that keeps most people healthy and free of suffering.

Liberalism and Rights

Social philosophy talked about duties but not rights until John Locke, the eighteenth-century British philosopher, emphasized the concept of natural rights. Locke's aim was to fight the tyranny of European governments and the vulnerability of the ordinary citizen, and the individual in general, to the unrestricted power of governments. He argued that human beings are born with **rights** attached to them by nature, including the right to freedom (autonomy), life, property ownership, and free expression. At that time, no such rights were granted except to the elite. Even the elite, other than the monarchs, were not allowed free expression in most circumstances. Citizens in Locke's time were granted limited rights through government decrees and statutes. These did not include the right to free speech or the pursuit of personal happiness.

In the Constitution of the United States, Americans were granted the right to life, liberty, and the pursuit of happiness. Additional rights, such as freedom of speech and to bear arms, were given later in the U.S. Bill of Rights. The notion of rights has advanced social and political philosophies to a large extent. In fact, the notions of human rights, equal civil rights, and freedom from oppression that dominated the twentieth century's movements of social and political reform were inspired by liberalism. The political aspect of liberalism is behind most of the principles of international law.

A right is defined as a valid claim. If a person is entitled to voting privileges and there are no sound legal reasons for denying this entitlement, he or she has a right (valid claim) to vote. This right allows him or her to expect other members of society not to interfere with his or her going to the polls and casting a vote. Rights, then, protect one's interests by imposing corresponding duties on other people to respect the interests of a right holder. In other words, every right has a corresponding duty on the part of other society members. Without such duty, exercising a right would be difficult. For example, your right to privacy cannot be exercised if your society does not consider it a duty to protect you from intruders. This is why no citizen in the former Soviet Union had a right to free speech: Citizens had no duty to help any person to express his or her opinions.

There are three important points about rights. First, rights differ from ordinary freedoms (privileges). For example, every person is entitled to play chess or to go to music concerts. But no person should expect others to help him or her play chess or go to concerts, because our society does not impose on us a duty to help other people enjoy freedoms. Yet every person expects others to help protect his or her property or privacy (either directly or by supporting the institutions that enforce law and order in society).

Second, there are moral rights and legal rights. Moral rights include the right to life, autonomy, and equality before the law. A moral right is a valid claim that is based on moral (ethical) reasons. For example, the right to life is based on the ethical principle that killing is wrong, and the right to autonomy is based on the principle that it is morally wrong to control other individuals. Although many moral rights are protected by law in most societies, some are not, so not every moral right is a legal right. Until the nineteenth century, for instance, slavery was legal in the U.S. The moral right to autonomy was not considered a legal right at that time.

At the same time, some legal rights may not be moral rights. For example, firing workers without significant compensation and when there is no economic need for reducing the workforce is a legal right for employers in the U.S. but not in Germany or Sweden. Germans and Swedes, among others, think that this right is based on an unfair principle that ignores the well being of workers. For an ethicist, the right of an employer to dismiss workers arbitrarily may seem difficult to accept on moral grounds, although it is allowed by law.

Third, rights are not absolute. They can be revoked or suspended. For example, a criminal is deprived of his right to autonomy when he is kept in jail. Similarly, the right to free speech is restricted by the rights of other people not to be defamed or slandered. It is true that people have the right to express their opinions, but it is also true that they should not misuse their rights and insult or humiliate others in the process.

Is liberalism relevant to health care ethics? Evidently, it enables medical ethics to utilize the concept of patients' rights and providers' corresponding duties to such rights. Without the concept of moral rights, which Locke called *natural rights*, it would be difficult to explore areas like privacy, confidentiality, informed consent, and paternalism. That will be seen more clearly in following chapters.

A right must not be confused with a **privilege.** As stated previously, a right is guaranteed for all persons. But privileges are not guaranteed (though not denied) for any person. No individual is entitled to claim the privilege of owning an expensive car or obtaining a license to practice dental hygiene. These privileges must be earned by effort and hard work. They are not guaranteed to whoever wants them. If a person wants to practice dental hygiene, he or she has to meet certain conditions required for licensure. Compare that with the right to life, for example. The right to life cannot be withheld and does not require hard work to be earned. It is guaranteed for all.

Controversies have arisen in the U.S. as to whether health care (including dental hygiene care) is a right for all residents or a privilege for those who can afford it through personal wealth or the ability to pay for insurance. And, if health care is ever guaranteed for all citizens, which benefits and procedures would be granted to every person who needs them? Would every treatment modality, regardless of its cost, be made available to all citizens who would benefit from them? Another controversy is education. Should post-secondary education be a privilege only for those who can afford the tuition? These are just a few examples that help distinguishing privilege from right.

Rawls's Theory of Justice

John Rawls is a contemporary American philosopher whose main concern has been social justice. He proposed a theory in the early 1970s that characterizes social justice as a fair deal that members of society negotiate and abide by (Rawls, 1971).

Contrary to the utilitarian view of justice as a means for happiness, Rawls asserts that justice is an end in itself. It is a situation that rational members of society desire and aspire to attain. Therefore, its principles cannot be arbitrary. These principles should be carefully sought and formulated. Meanwhile, the principles of justice cannot be reached by speculation that fails to consider the real wants and needs of people in society. If philosophers introduce principles of justice that are theoretically elegant and admirable but practically unrealizable or unacceptable to the average person, these principles will never work.

Rawls's idea is that people do not need a profound thinker to advise them about justice. Rather, they need to reach an agreement among themselves, based on rational debate, that they accept and enact. But to reach a lasting agreement, people need to think impartially. Our experience with modern science tells us that scientists agree easily on the same conclusions and interpretations of data because they think impartially. It may be true that practitioners of science, when they strictly follow the scientific method, can be impartial. But impartiality is more difficult to achieve in daily life, where various kinds of biased attitudes influence people.

Yet Rawls finds a way out. He believes that people will be impartial if they are ignorant about their personal status, economic situation, and social standing. The reason is that people will not be biased to a group, profession, or class if they have no idea about where they stand. Imagine that you do not know whether you will be a professional, a merchant, a skilled laborer, or a manual worker. Would you take sides with those who demand equal tax cuts for every citizen, so that the rich do not pay more than the poor? Or with those who advocate raising minimum wage? Perhaps you would be rather neutral on both issues. But a low-income worker would typically side with the latter issue, while an owner of a corporation would side with the former. This seems acceptable because people tend to favor the proposals and plans that serve their own interests. This assumption that people act from self-interest underlies Rawls's theory.

Rawls calls the situation in which people can be impartial the *original position*. In this imaginary situation, people would discuss justice with (to speak metaphorically) a veil of ignorance in front of their eyes. Only in this situation, Rawls believes, could people think without preconceived biases and therefore reach reasonable agreements. His line of reasoning is that people think, argue, and act from self-interest. If someone knew that he or she would be a nuclear physicist, that person would believe that it is just to reward people with intellectual abilities. If the same person knew that he or she would be a factory worker, he or she would think that people should be rewarded according to the physical effort they expend to produce goods. However, if people were in the original position, they would agree on a system of principles that causes the least harm to any of them if they turn out to be in the least privileged class or group.

Rawls supposes (with good reasons) that in the original position, people would agree on principles that promote mutual self-interest and that they would not agree except on principles that further the interests of them all. Thus self-interest in combination with rational thinking would impose a cautious attitude. Rational, self-interested people would not take risks; they would be careful. They would not assume that they might eventually be in the elite class, so in order to avoid harming themselves if they happen to be in a lower position, they would not choose principles that favor the top class. Rawls assumes that ignorance about one's future position would suppress the gambling, irrational attitude in people and would motivate them to think cautiously. In other words, they would be primarily guided by risk aversion.

Self-interest, moreover, would guide people to insist on equal basic liberties for all. Such liberties include free speech, autonomy, equal opportunities, and similar essential freedoms. Not many people, in Rawls's opinion, would be willing to sacrifice these badly needed liberties. Self-interest would also direct them to prefer abundance with some degree of inequality to equality with scarcity, because satisfying basic needs comes before the need for fairness, at least for most people. As Rawls sees it, any person would prefer to have a big piece of a large pie that is cut into unequal but sizable pieces rather than a tiny piece of a smaller pie that is cut into exactly equal pieces (so that every person gets an equal share). That is, Rawls thinks that every reasonable person would say, "I want to eat enough, no matter how much the other guy is eating." What Rawls wants to conclude here is that justice cannot be absolute and that the demand for justice is restricted by other factors, particularly by the need for abundance.

It follows that if the motivation to work productively (which is essential for affluence) requires inequality (which will result from rewarding productive more than nonproductive people), it would be reasonable to allow the least possible degree of inequality required for increasing productivity. Based on this situation, people will conclude that justice can be established on two basic principles, which are commonly called Rawls's two principles of justice.

The first principle says that each person has an equal right to the most extensive scheme of equal basic liberties that a society can afford. These liberties should be guaranteed for each person to the extent that they do not undermine the liberties of others. That is, no person can have a degree of liberty which, for being too much, decreases the amounts of liberties available to others (and consequently leads to inequality).

The second principle says that social and economic goods may be distributed unequally under two conditions. First, these inequalities should work for the benefit of the least advantaged. Second, they should be made open to fair competition in which all members of society can participate. All precautions must be taken to ensure that any person can fairly compete for advantaged positions. That is, these privileged positions must be given only to those who deserve them, not to members of an elite or favored class.

Why should the least advantaged be favored? This is an important question that poses itself at this point. Rawls's answer is that inequality is not a prize given to the gifted to express our admiration. It is a "carrot" to tempt the gifted to do their best for others. This is not an exploitation of the gifted, though. A gifted person may argue that hard work, not merely talent, earned him or her success. However, the motivation to work hard is determined by a personal quality that is derived from genes. What comes from nature is a resource, like water and minerals, and resources are liable to fair distribution. Unequal income, then, is not naturally deserved by the gifted but was granted them in a deal that was negotiated in the original, hypothetical, position. Less gifted people chose to allow for such a privilege (which they could have chosen not to grant to the gifted) in return for a commitment by the gifted to pay back.

Rawls would, for example, say, "If you are an excellent entrepreneur while I am an ordinary person, I still have some right to your achievements because your intelligence is an asset like other natural resources. If your talent does not work for my advantage, you have done injustice to me because your talent (like oil wells or rivers) should be used for everyone's benefit." So, according to Rawls's theory, the talented should realize that they have already entered an agreement in the original position to work first for the least advantaged. If they change their minds after becoming privileged, they should be reminded of their initial judgment and agreement, which was made when impartiality was possible (i.e., under the veil of ignorance).

How does this theory fit into the problems addressed by health care ethics? Remember that health care goods are limited while the needs for them are immense. That is, there is a relative but significant scarcity of health care resources. These resources need to be distributed carefully. Should we allow the rich to have the best resources for themselves because they can afford to pay for them? Utilitarians disagree, because favoring the rich, or any particular section of society, limits the general happiness to this section alone and lets the suffering of other sections grow. The ultimate result is a reduction in the total happiness in society, which is morally undesirable. But Rawls rejects tying justice to happiness. Yet he reaches the same utilitarian conclusion: Health care resources should be distributed fairly among all members of society. How does he justify this answer? Recall the original position. If people are in that position, which is conducive to impartiality, they would choose the arrangement that exposes them to the least risk. Since none of them know whether they will be healthy or ill, able to pay medical bills or unable even to buy necessary medication, they would choose a system that makes the most privileged responsible to work for improving the situation of the least advantaged.

Reflect on the conclusions of utilitarianism and Rawls's theory. Both favor an arrangement that ensures that all, or at least most, people get equal access to basic health care services (e.g., emergency care and immunizations) and almost equal access to every other form of essential health care service. Utilitarians want that arrangement to increase the happiness in the world, and Rawls wants it because it agrees with people's attitudes and inclinations, at least when they think impartially. A system of national health insurance would be ideal for both philosophies, although any system that guarantees affordable care for every member of society would be acceptable to them.

Ideally, every person should have access to any form of health care that he or she needs. But the scarcity of resources imposes practical restrictions on distributing healthcare services and necessitates drawing a distinction, however arbitrary, between "badly needed" and "less urgently needed" services. Unfortunately, not all dental care or preventive dental hygiene care is considered "needed" health care in terms of insurance or government assistance programs (see Chapter 6, "Social Issues"). Let us hope that future advances in technology succeed in reducing the cost of health care.

SUMMARY

The discipline of ethics consists of thoughts and ideas about morality. The study of normative ethics can be divided into two major groups of theories: deontology and teleology (consequentialism). Deontological theories (Kant's ethics) emphasize duties, while teleological theories emphasize consequences of actions. Utilitarianism is a teleological theory concerned with attaining the greatest amount of utility, usefulness, or happiness. Social philosophy is concerned mainly with rights of people and social justice. A right is a valid claim and is ensured for all people. A privilege, by contrast, is not guaranteed and must be attained by personal effort or optional help from people who want to provide such help. Although no person is obligated to help others attain a privilege, there is no moral rule that forbids volunteering to help someone to gain a privilege in a way that does not harm others. Utilitarians view social justice as a means to happiness and, for this reason, they pursue justice. Because utilitarianism considers justice a moral goal, it recommends that society allocate goods and services, such as health care resources, in a fair way.

SELF-TEST

1. Utilitarianism is concerned with
    a) rights
    b) duties
    c) happiness
    d) total amount of happiness in the world
    e) privileges
2. Kantian ethics is concerned with
    a) rights
    b) duties
    c) happiness
    d) total amount of happiness in the world
    e) privileges

3. Utilitarians are concerned with consequences when making ethical decisions.
   a) True
   b) False
4. If person *A* has a *right,* then person *B* has a *duty* to ensure that right.
   a) True
   b) False
5. A *privilege* is granted only if certain conditions are met.
   a) True
   b) False
6. A deontological approach would look at the benefit or happiness that would result from a decision, while a teleological approach would not consider the consequences.
   a) True
   b) False

ACTIVITIES

1. Divide into groups. Relate to one another situations in which decisions had to be made. Classify the decisions based on the ethical theories or approaches. Present these findings to the class. Does the class agree with your classifications?
2. Design a case study or scenario that would involve a decision that a dental hygienist may have to make regarding patient care or a public health need. Select an ethical theory. Defend the decision using the selected ethical theory.

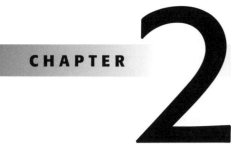

CHAPTER

2

Ethical Principles and Core Values

OBJECTIVES

Upon reading the material in this chapter, you will be able to

1. Identify the core values found in the Code of Ethics of the American Dental Hygienists' Association.
2. Define the terms autonomy, confidentiality, societal trust, non-maleficence, beneficence, justice, veracity, fidelity, paternalism, and utility.

INTRODUCTION

Decisions and actions of health care providers are guided by ethical principles and core values. These core values are based on the Hippocratic Oath and similar codes (see Appendix A). They have evolved through the years as professions formulate their own individual codes of ethics. Core values are selected ethical principles that are considered central to a particular code of ethics (see Table 2–1). In the Code of Ethics of the American Dental Hygienists' Association (ADHA), seven core values are identified: autonomy, confidentiality, societal trust, nonmaleficence, beneficence, justice, and veracity (Table 2–1).

Table 2-1 Core Values of the ADHA Code of Ethics

Value	Description
Autonomy	to guarantee self-determination of the patient
Confidentiality	to hold in confidence or secret information entrusted by the patient
Societal Trust	to ensure the trust patients and society have in dental hygienists
Nonmaleficence	to do no harm to the patient
Beneficence	to benefit the patient
Justice	to be fair to the patient; fairness
Veracity	to tell the truth; not to lie to the patient

ETHICAL PRINCIPLES

Autonomy

Autonomy is *self-determination.* An autonomous person controls his or her own actions, behavior, and inner life (i.e., plans, goals, convictions, and beliefs). He or she also decides which values to advocate, which faith to adhere to, and which life styles to adopt. As seen in Chapter 1, "Introduction to Moral Philosophy and Moral Reasoning," the Kantian principle of respect for persons implies that every individual should be valued and appreciated. It follows that the preferences of every person should be respected by fellow human beings. This is how the Kantian principle substantiates the concept of autonomy. The right to autonomy is among the fundamental rights emphasized by libertarian philosophers and proponents of human rights. Although the right to autonomy began as a moral right, that is, a right that morality calls for, it soon became an essential component of our legal rights.

Individuals, then, should be able to decide for themselves what actions they will take, even if these seem foolish to others. There are limits to autonomy. People are free to behave as they choose, only as long as they do not harm others. Indeed, harm is the main restriction on autonomy. Fortunately, we can all be autonomous without harming each other because it is easy for rational persons to consider the interests of other persons and to act in a way that preserves them.

What are the implications of autonomy for health care? If competent adults are granted the right to autonomy, they should be permitted to accept or refuse any actions that affect their lives. Consequently, competent patients (and guardians or parents of incompetent patients) should be allowed to accept or refuse treatment. Some patients have limited knowledge of health-related issues and therefore cannot decide upon a proposed treatment unless they are informed about its effectiveness, cost, likelihood of success, side effects, and so on. As a result, it is the right of a patient to have adequate information about an action, such as an operation, that will affect his or her life. With this information, the person can agree to a treatment plan or refuse it. This is precisely how the notion of informed consent, which is discussed in the next chapter, is derived from the right to autonomy.

The ADHA Code of Ethics emphasizes the core value of individual autonomy and the rights that follow from it: "People have the right to be treated with respect. They have the right to informed consent prior to treatment, and they have the right to full disclosure of all relevant information so that they can make informed choices about their care" (ADHA, 1999, p. 17).

Confidentiality

Confidentiality is the avoidance of revealing any personal information about the patient. Personal information may be sensitive or even embarrassing, and failure to keep it within proper bounds can harm the patient in various ways. The practice of keeping private information about patients confidential should extend to all kinds of personal information, not just to shameful or embarrassing information.

Confidentiality differs from privacy in that confidentiality involves a promise from a trusted person. If a person entrusts a friend, for example, not to publicize personal information, the friend implicitly promises to keep the information confidential. Similarly, patients giving their providers personal information about themselves assume that the providers are implicitly promising confidentiality. Keeping a promise is a moral duty that every ethical theory emphasizes, so it would be unethical of providers to reveal any personal information relevant to their patients. Confidentiality is also a legal duty of health care providers and a patient's right (see Chapter 5, "Jurisprudence").

It is true that patients who voluntarily give personal information to their providers are, in effect, giving up their right to privacy. The act of sharing information itself implies declining the right to privacy. But the right to privacy also includes the right to determine what will be shared with whom. Consequently, individuals declining their right to privacy by sharing personal information with providers do not lose their right to determine whether any other individual can have access to this information. Thus the provider cannot pass any personal information to any party without permission from the patient.

Unfortunately, in this age of computers and information technology, confidentiality is harder to maintain. Health care information is available not only to the health care providers but also to any individual who has access to medical records, such as employees of health insurance companies. Yet a careful provider would not keep sensitive information on records that can be made available to others.

As already pointed out, confidentiality may be breached if there is a moral justification for disclosure or if the patient requests or consents to the disclosure. For example, one may disclose confidential information in certain cases to another healthcare provider if the information is relevant to helping the patient. Circumstances that allow for disclosing confidential information include:

1. An emergency.
2. To protect third parties.
3. When required by law (e.g., sexually transmitted disease, child or elderly abuse).
4. When requesting commitment or hospitalization of a mentally ill patient.
   (Purtilo, 1999, p. 154; Guitheil & Applebaum, 1988).

A hypothetical example for an emergency in dental hygiene practice would be the following. A patient experiences chest pain in the dental chair and you call for an ambulance. You remember that the patient told you that he abuses cocaine, and you have documented this in the medical history. Knowing that cocaine can induce severe, potentially fatal heart disease, you reveal to the paramedics upon their arrival the information about your patient's substance abuse. Normally, no information from a patient's health history can be relayed to another provider without the patient signing a release form.

In this case, however, the information you give the paramedics will help in the diagnosis and treatment of the present chest pains and potential heart problem. Breach of confidentiality may occasionally be necessary to protect a third party. For example, a patient has more severe attrition on his teeth than on his last visit. He states that he grinds his teeth more since his divorce because he is still angry with his wife. He tells you that he will one day kill his wife for what she has done to him. Here you have an obligation to protect her by contacting her or the police, because you know that threats made by emotionally upset people can be serious.

Societal Trust

Trust is another core value that is incorporated into the ADHA Code of Ethics. The Code states, "We value client trust and understand that public trust in our profession is based on our actions and behavior" (ADHA, 1999, p. 17). The public, as individual patients and society in general, acknowledges dental hygienists' possession of specialized knowledge and skill. It is our ethical duty to ensure that this trust is maintained. However, this may be difficult when society views health care providers as concerned with their self-interest more than with the patients' interests. Society may form such a view when they suspect that providers act as "gatekeepers" for "for-profit" companies such as health care management organizations. In fact, many individuals believe that the present system has turned providers into employees eager to serve insurance companies and other employers more than they are interested in serving their patients. As a profession that values and relies on societal trust, dental hygiene must be alert to such misconceptions and must resist any attempt by for-profit organizations to endanger the interests of patients for financial gain.

Societal trust can also be jeopardized if the public perceives a breach of confidentiality. This is why dental hygienists and other providers should avoid providing any confidential information about their patients to a third party. If any practical need for revealing such information to a third party emerges, providers should weigh the benefit and cost of revealing. It may happen, for example, that the authorities investigating a crime request access to records of some patients, or that HIV-positive patients admit to their providers unprotected sexual behavior. In such situations, protecting the interests of society override the right to confidentiality. But there may be less obvious situations that are more difficult to judge. To deal with situations of this sort, the provider must examine two questions. First, is the harm of threatening societal trust in the profession outweighed by the benefit of revealing confidential information? Second, how can the amount of harm be kept to a minimum when it becomes ethically appropriate to break a confidence. (Purtilo, 1999, p.156).

Nonmaleficence

Nonmaleficence means to *do no harm* to others. Although the principle of doing no harm may not always seem sufficient for guiding human behavior, it is the most basic element in morality. In other words, it is a necessary condition for morality. If an action involves harming a person or a group, it cannot be considered moral. However, as already pointed out, there are situations that require providing tangible help for other people. For example, it is ethical not to interfere with the efforts of the Red Cross that are intended to relieve a famine in Africa. By not protesting or denouncing such efforts, or by merely acknowledging them, one is demonstrating *nonmaleficence.* But suppose a person knows that the resources of the Red Cross and similar organizations are too limited to feed the hundreds of thousands that are dying of hunger. Would that person be acting morally by doing nothing other than approving of the good will of these organizations? In fact, a person who has a genuine interest in morality would feel compelled to participate in the effort of shipping or distributing food or donating money for famine relief. That is, by not doing anything, one may be doing harm.

Both beneficence and nonmaleficence are among the principles emphasized by the Hippocratic Oath, although nonmaleficence is stressed as the most basic principle. The Oath says *primum non nocere:* First, do no harm. More recent codes of ethics that are adopted by healthcare professions also deal with nonmaleficence as the foundation for medical ethics. The ADHA Code of Ethics states "We accept our fundamental obligation to provide services in a manner that protects all clients and minimizes harm to them and others involved in their treatment" (ADHA, 1999, p. 17). In practice, dental hygienists act ethically when they apply all the measures that prevent harm, such as the universal precautions and thorough debridement. These two examples also demonstrate adherence to "standard of care," which is closely related to nonmaleficence. Standard of care is discussed in Chapter 5, "Jurisprudence."

Beneficence

Beneficence means doing what will *benefit* a person (for example, a patient). Most ethical thinkers feel that doing no harm to other people (nonmaleficence) is not sufficient in all situations. A person who wants to do what is morally right will often find it necessary to offer active help to others. As dental hygienists, according to the ADHA Code of Ethics, we have "a primary role in promoting the well being of individuals and the public by engaging in health promotion/disease prevention activities" (ADHA, 1999, p. 17). This is consistent with the Report of the Surgeon General, which emphasizes that "oral health is essential to the general health and well-being of all Americans *and* can be achieved by all Americans (U.S. Department of Health and Human Services, 2000, p. 1). Thus, dental hygienists, as members of a profession that is meant to help the public, have obligations that extend beyond individual patients to society as a whole. In fact, societies have developed health care professions, including dental hygiene, to benefit their members. The principle of beneficence therefore underlies our profession.

Dental hygienists are becoming more involved in public service and do not limit their efforts to providing care for private patients. They manage and operate programs in rural and remote areas and offer care to residents of nursing homes and geriatric facilities. Many hygienists also volunteer in preventive projects that are intended to help members of their communities, particularly of the less privileged. Fluoridation programs are examples for these projects. Such contributions to society show that the profession of dental hygiene is primarily guided by the principle of beneficence. Another form of beneficence is *pro bono,* which is donating one's services. A dental hygienist who donates time and skills to a public clinic or who arranges with the employer to treat those unable to pay is practicing the ethical principle of beneficence.

Justice

Justice can be defined as *fairness.* In the ADHA Code of Ethics, justice and fairness are considered together as one core value. The code states, "We value justice and support the fair and equitable distribution of health care resources. We believe all people should have access to high-quality, affordable oral health care" (ADHA, 1999, p. 17). This position is concerned with individual and social groups. It emphasizes that patients should receive the same quality of care regardless of their socioeconomic status, ethnicity, education, or ability to pay. The concept of justice has been discussed in Chapter 1, "Introduction to Moral Philosophy and Moral Reasoning," and will be discussed further in Chapter 6, "Social Issues."

Veracity

Veracity is telling the *truth.* According to the code, "We accept our obligation to tell the truth and assume that others will do the same. We value self-knowledge and seek truth and honesty in all relationships." (ADHA, 1999, p. 17). Truthfulness is a very important component in professional ethics. It is often in the best interest of the patient to know about his or her condition. Partial disclosure may lead to false hopes or unnecessary despair. Incomplete information, such as not telling patients of a less expensive option for treatment, may also generate financial or practical problems for patients. More importantly, withholding truth from patients can threaten the trust between the patient and provider. As discussed in Chapter 3, "Informed Consent," full disclosure of pertinent information is important for informed consent. Veracity and "gag clauses" will be further discussed in Chapter 6, "Social Issues."

Occasionally, a health care provider finds that withholding truth would serve the patient's interests more than truthfulness. In that case, it may be justified not to be truthful with the patient, at least temporarily. This kind of "therapeutic deception" is referred to as the *therapeutic privilege*. However, this practice should be limited to cases that definitely require it. Telling a patient that local anesthesia will eliminate any discomfort may be deception if the patient is not also told that pressure will be felt or that there may be discomfort as the anesthesia wears off. Telling a child that dental treatment will not hurt, when in fact it may, or telling an adult that the only treatment option is the one covered by insurance, when in fact there are other options, are both examples of deception.

Fidelity

Fidelity is an ethical responsibility closely related to veracity, trust, and confidentiality. Fidelity means that the health care provider will be *faithful* to promises and obligations, will abide by rules and regulations, and will meet all reasonable expectations. Also, fidelity means that the health care provider will act as a fiduciary, or a person who will act in the best interest of the patient. Although fidelity is not listed as a core value in the ADHA Code of Ethics, it is implied by other explicitly stated principles, such as trust and veracity.

Paternalism/Parentalism

The terms **parentalism** and **paternalism** are used synonymously to denote acting like a parent with the intent to protect or enhance the interests of a person at a time when that person is unable or unwilling to protect his or her own interests. In such a situation, the autonomy of the protected person is restricted and his or her freedom of choice is ignored or suppressed. The most acceptable form of paternalism is practicing natural parenthood, where parents do what is in the best interest of their children. Paternalism becomes a problem when the person on whose behalf another person is acting is a competent adult. Because competent adults can know what is useful or harmful for them, they need no other person to decide on their behalf. Indeed, a person who volunteers to make good decisions for competent adults would be violating that adult's autonomy.

Does it follow that every act of paternalism is wrong? Suppose that a nurse saw a person in the clinic suffering from low blood pressure and circulatory collapse. He or she thinks that this patient needs urgent admission to the hospital to save his or her life, but the patient refuses. It is apparent that his or her refusal is the result of poor circulation, which causes impaired judgment and mental confusion. Should the nurse make a paternalistic decision and send the patient to the hospital without delay, despite his or her protest? One is inclined to say yes, but it is difficult to justify forcing people to get treatment when they do not want to. However, knowing that acute illness frequently impairs the capacity to think soundly seems to be a good reason for an exceptional violation of autonomy. Furthermore, the nurse is not infringing on the patient's autonomy except to preserve the right to life. In normal circumstances, the patient would readily accept admission for treatment. So emergencies and temporary impairment of judgment may validate paternalistic actions on behalf of competent adults. Most well-intentioned paternalistic acts towards incompetent patients and patients that are considered minors are justifiable.

In dentistry, a patient may be told what a treatment will be and not be given a choice. For example, a dentist may decide what type of material and procedure will be used for a restoration without telling the patient the other options for restorative treatment. By telling the patient only what the dentist feels the patient needs to know and by withholding other information, the dentist has made a paternal decision and has violated the autonomy of the patient.

In many situations, paternalism is not practiced by individuals but by institutions or governments. There are, for example, laws that prohibit the use of recreational drugs with the intent to protect people—even competent adults—from addiction and consequential hazards. In most states, the law requires all drivers and passengers to wear seat belts to protect them from injury in traffic accidents. Both examples reflect paternalistic settings, where the state is acting on behalf of citizens to protect their interests. Yet some competent citizens do not want that protection and feel that they should be allowed to choose whether or not they use drugs or fasten seat belts. The state seems to such individuals an oppressive agency that restricts their freedom and denies their autonomy. However, the consequences of addiction and serious accidents are not limited to the individuals who chose to harm themselves. Society shares the cost incurred by the unsound choices that some of its members make. It would be justified, at least for this reason, to accept particular forms of institutional (impersonal) paternalism. In fact, the most obvious form of institutional paternalism in the U.S. is the Food and Drug Administration (FDA). This agency decides for us which drugs are safe and which are risky. It limits our freedom of choice but at the same time protects us from potential harm. In public dental health programs, water fluoridation benefits the public and protects against caries. However, some citizens feel that this is forcing fluoride on individuals and may even be detrimental to the public's health.

Utility

Utility, or the *usefulness* of an action, underlies the theory of utilitarianism (see Chapter 1, "Introduction to Moral Philosophy and Moral Reasoning"). The utility principle encompasses beneficence and nonmaleficence, but goes beyond them. It is needed because neither beneficence nor nonmaleficence alone can solve the conflicts and competing needs in society. Suppose, for example, that a group of dental hygienists want to help the elderly poor in rural areas of their county to get sufficient preventive care. Guided by beneficence, the group considers sending three hygienists each week to a different remote area to take care of its elderly residents, but the funds they are able to raise will not cover all the expenses of the project. Some suggest transferring part of a fund that is intended for serving patients in county nursing homes. Others disagree because the needs of urban nursing-home residents are equal to those of rural residents. In such a situation, beneficence alone cannot tell the hygienists whether any group deserves more funds than the other. It can only tell them that it is morally good to help both groups. Similarly, nonmaleficence would not offer the needed answer. But the utility principle can be a reliable guide in that context.

The principle of utility is required to assess and rank the needs and wants of individuals or groups and to help determine social priorities. It can offer answers to questions about how to allocate resources and how to deal with the various needs of different sectors of society without causing significant harm to any sector. In effect, the principle imposes a social duty on us all to use our resources to do as much good as possible. That is, we must do the most good overall, even when this means we are not able to meet all needs in a particular area (Munson, 1999, p. 36).

When health care providers confront important decisions, they should consider the benefits and burdens of each available choice. They should try to realize the greatest benefit and the least harm for their patients and community. The utility principle is useful not only for making choices and decisions regarding issues pertaining to groups but also for issues that concern individuals. For example, this principle can guide us to determine whether the risk of a diagnostic test outweighs the benefit of the information it provides.

SUMMARY

Professional ethical behavior is guided by ethical principles and core values found in codes of ethics. The Code of Ethics of the ADHA identifies seven core values: autonomy, confidentiality, societal trust, nonmaleficence, beneficence, justice, and veracity. Other ethical principles include justified paternalism, utility, and fidelity. In some situations these values conflict with each other, leading to ethical dilemmas. The right of patients to autonomy (i.e., to decide for themselves how they can be treated) should be respected by health care providers. However, in specific circumstances, this right may be restricted for the patient's benefit (e.g., with incompetent patients and in emergencies).

SELF-TEST

1. Match the following terms with definitions:

   ___ Justice   A. Truth-telling
   ___ Beneficence   B. Fairness
   ___ Fidelity   C. Benefiting others
   ___ Nonmaleficence   D. No harm
   ___ Veracity   E. Faithfulness

2. Confidentiality is an important core value, or ethical principle. Why?

3. Beneficence means
   a) to do what is good for yourself
   b) truth-telling
   c) to do what is good for others
   d) faithfulness

4. Nonmaleficence means
   a) to do no harm
   b) to do only what is beneficial
   c) to tell the truth
   d) to do only the harm that the patient accepts

5. Justice is a core principle found in a code of ethics. It means ____ in treating patients.
   a) applying the law strictly
   b) fairness
   c) fair paternalism
   d) doing equal harm or benefit

6. Truth-telling is the core value or ethical principle of _____.
    a) veracity
    b) honesty
    c) frankness
    d) virtuousness

7. Avoidance of disseminating private information about patients is _____.

8. Veracity and fairness cannot be applied simultaneously in the same situation.
    a) True
    b) False

ACTIVITIES

1. Develop a code of ethics for dental hygiene students to follow while treating patients and interacting with fellow students and faculty.
2. Compare the newly developed code of ethics with the ADHA Code of Ethics.
3. Report on a situation that you encountered in clinic where you were forced to make a decision between conflicting actions. Determine which core values or ethical principles were involved.

CASE STUDY

Contributed by Debi Gerger, RDH, BS, MPH Program/Clinic Coordinator, San Joaquin Valley College, Rancho Cucamonga, CA.

Scenario: You have recently been hired as a dental hygienist in a progressive general practice. The dentist appears very nice and professional and has offered you three days per week with a satisfying salary. After working in the office for one week, the dentist asks you to begin utilizing the intraoral camera when doing assessments. You feel confident and comfortable with the camera; therefore this request does not seem to be a problem. The dentist then states that you are required to use the camera only for obvious problem areas, but you are to find four problem areas in each adult patient at each recall visit. These problems are to be placed on the video monitor for the patient to see and to enable the dental hygienist to educate the patient. This procedure is to facilitate the exam process for the dentist. In analyzing this case, consider which of the ethical principles are involved. Recognize that this case involves the dental hygienist, the dentist, and the patient.

Discussion: One of the first items that you should be concerned about is why the dentist is requiring you to find four items on each adult patient recall visit. Does the dentist want you to be more thorough with your assessment? Does the dentist want the exam to go more quickly and smoothly? Does the dentist want to increase production? What if you found more than four problem areas?

Many of the ethical principles discussed in this chapter can be applied to this case study. The first principle that may come to mind is *trust*. The public trusts our profession to provide skilled and competent care. In this case, the patient trusts the problem areas you found with the camera are indeed problems that need attention. When pushed to find four problems in each adult patient, the dental hygienist may have to be deceptive in his or her communication with the patient.

Another principle to consider in this situation is *veracity.* Honesty is an integral part of the profession and cannot be jeopardized. In this case study, there may be occasions that the dental hygienist will be truthful, but there will also be occasions when it is impossible to be truthful.

It is simple to use the intraoral camera, but it is not so simple to ignore the dentist's request. What will you do?

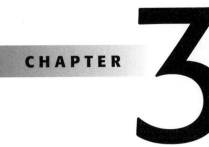

INFORMED CONSENT

OBJECTIVES

Upon reading the material in this chapter, you will be able to

1. Discuss the criteria necessary for informed consent.
2. Relate conditions for *not* obtaining informed consent.
3. Compare the ethical principles found in codes of ethics, informed consent, patients' bills of rights, and other documents related to patient care.

INTRODUCTION

Informed consent is the patient's acceptance of a line of treatment based on the information provided by a health care provider. Simply, there are two sides to informed consent: being *informed* and giving *consent*. That is, the patient is provided sufficient information about his or her condition and the available treatment options. Then the patient is allowed to discuss these options with the provider and to choose the most suitable treatment alternative.

The notion of informed consent was narrow and restricted until a few decades ago when some court decisions triggered interest in reexamining and widening this notion. In the past, informed consent consisted of a patient signing, before surgery, a form stating the name of the operation and the risks associated with it. The purpose of these forms was two-fold: telling the patient about the nature of the procedure and its advantages and risks, and ensuring legal protection for the practitioner if one of the mentioned risks occurs. That context seemed ethical enough at the time. After all, the practitioner was acting ethically by doing what was *right* for the patient (i.e., what he or she considered to be in the best interest of the patient). At present, the concept of informed consent is understood not merely as obtaining documented consent from a patient. Rather, it is considered a well-intended discussion between a provider and patient, informing the patient about every relevant aspect in the proposed procedure, the alternative procedures, and the points that the patient should consider while opting for a particular procedure. That is, the provider is no longer an authority who decides what is best for the patient.

At first thought, the concept of informed consent may seem easy to understand: A practitioner tells the patient what will be performed and the patient agrees. But on further consideration, several initially unexplored aspects begin to appear. To what extent should the patient be informed? Should the explanations offered to patients involve technical details? Should the uncommon adverse effects of a therapeutic modality be specified? Would a practitioner be legally protected if he or she warns patients that the probability of the elected procedure causing severe bleeding is only 1 in 300, then a patient happens to bleed excessively from that procedure? Could the failure of obtaining an informed consent automatically free the practitioner of legal liability if the patient's health deteriorates due to his or her decision to withhold treatment? These are only a few examples of countless questions surrounding informed consent. In fact, the concept of informed consent is multidimensional and involves substantial legal and moral issues.

It may appear that by the mere action of entering your operatory, a patient is demonstrating consent, for if the patient had at least second thoughts about receiving your treatment, he or she would not be there. Yet this patient is likely to be demonstrating trust in a provider rather than consent. Meanwhile, not every consent is an informed consent. Patients should clearly know exactly what they are consenting to and what they can expect from the offered choice of treatment. They ought to be also told about possible hazards and adverse effects. Moreover, patients' actions that demonstrate trust in their provider must not be interpreted as consent. The importance of a clear and concise explanation of the treatment plan so that both the dental hygienist and the patient know what is expected at each appointment cannot be overemphasized.

RIGHTS AND DUTIES INVOLVED IN INFORMED CONSENT

So far, it has been implied that patients have a right to be informed and to make an independent decision whether to accept or reject a procedure or treatment strategy. Recall the discussion of rights in Chapter 1, "Introduction to Moral Philosophy and Moral Reasoning." We have seen that people have basic rights, which include the right to life, autonomy, and fair treatment. Where would the right to informed consent be placed? The answer is that this right is a derivative one. It is derived from the right to autonomy. If patients are granted autonomy, that is, freedom of thought and action, they should be enabled to choose the alternative treatment modality that they find appropriate for the circumstance. But to do that, this patient should be helped to carefully evaluate the available modalities and select the most suitable one. As already discussed, every right has a corresponding duty. In this case, the patient's right to informed consent entails the duty of health care providers to adequately inform and advise the patient and the duty not to try to influence any decision for reasons other than the patient's best interest. This is how the issue of informed consent relates to ethics.

EVOLUTION OF THE CONCEPT OF INFORMED CONSENT

There are three basic forms of consent. The first is *implied consent*. Patients opening their mouths for examinations without actually stating or signing forms saying that they agree to be examined are communicating an implied consent to the providers. Although they do not explicitly state their consent, they act as if they agree to be examined by the providers. The second form of consent is *expressed consent*, in which the patient verbally agrees to a recommended procedure. The third form is *written consent,* where the patient signs a statement authorizing the provider to perform a suggested procedure. For all these forms of consent to be ethical and legal, the patient must be informed about the procedure and must have the opportunity to comprehend and evaluate the risks and benefits of the suggested treatment (Wilkins, 1999, p. 328).

The Hippocratic Oath and Code of Ethics, which is intended for health professionals, emphasizes the ethical principles of *beneficence* (doing what will benefit the patient) and *nonmaleficence* (doing no harm). Historically, practitioners made decisions on the basis of benefiting and not harming the patient. This practice, which is as old as the dawn of the art of healing, implied that physicians (or healers) act from benevolence towards their patients and that patients, in return, entrust them with their lives. Consent in that context was not really informed, but based on faith in the competence and dedication of the practitioner, that is, a belief that the practitioner knows best what should be done to treat each patient. In other words, informing patients was regarded as redundant and therefore not a right that patients were entitled to. So, the idea of informed consent is relatively new.

In modern times, societies introduced measures to protect patients from unfounded trust in their health care providers. They introduced elaborate systems of licensing and assessing the competency of professionals. However, the "beneficence-nonmaleficence" practice continued to govern the relationship between patients and health care providers. This construal of consent as trust-dependent was the basis of the *harm-avoidance model* of informed consent, which was introduced many decades ago. In this model there is an obvious underestimation of the duty to inform the patient adequately; it has recently been modified. The reluctance of physicians and other practitioners in the past, when the harmavoidance model was still popular, to disclose information is possibly explained by the following *assumptions* that health professionals made.

1. Patients do not want to know or to participate in making decisions about their treatment. Perhaps it is true that some did not want to, but it would be wrong to generalize.
2. Patients would not understand the information anyway.
3. The physician/provider always knows what is in the best interest of the patient, making it unnecessary to get the patient involved and further complicate matters.
4. The physician/provider has both the authority and appropriate medical knowledge to prescribe certain treatments to the patient, who has an obligation not to dispute their validity.
5. Patients are, in most instances, extremely uninformed about their health, which makes it rather tedious, costly, and time consuming for providers to discuss treatment in any detail (Switankowsky, 1998, p. 37).

Therefore, in the harm-avoidance model the practitioner adopts *paternalism* or *parentalism,* or the attitude of acting like a parent who knows what is best for the patient, and the patient accepts that. As you may recall from our earlier discussion of the concept of paternalism, autonomy and paternalism do not go together. Indeed, paternalism infringes on autonomy.

Another drawback inherent in this model is that it encourages, or at least justifies, deceiving patients in order to motivate them or enhance their compliance. For example, a practitioner who hopes to benefit and protect a cancer patient may tell the patient that he or she has a chronic benign disease so that the patient does not abandon treatment out of despair or refuse a major surgery that could slow down his or her cancer. Similarly, a physician may give false information to his or her patient, either explicitly or by hinting about a prognosis of the severe disease, to protect the patient from depression and anxiety. In the former example, the provider ignored, even denied, the *patient's right* to decide whether he or she wanted radical therapy or merely symptomatic relief. In the latter example, the provider denied the patient's right to decide which practical arrangements he or she needs or wishes to make before dying (e.g., paying debt or modifying a will). In both examples, the providers acted from seemingly moral and legitimate principles. They were literally applying the beneficence and nonmaleficence principles. To accomplish their seemingly ethical goal (i.e., keeping their patients healthy for as long as possible), they ignored the patients' wishes and thought that it was justifiable to deceive them. But this paternalistic attitude toward informed consent, which permits the provider to determine which information is to be conveyed to or withheld from the patient, is no longer accepted. As can be easily seen, paternalism ascribes unlimited authority to the provider and restricts the autonomy of the patient. Nonetheless, as will be shown, there are exceptional situations in which it is morally acceptable to hide information from certain patients.

The current, more recent concept of informed consent is referred to as the *autonomy-enhancing model.* It has replaced the harm-avoidance model. This model acknowledges the patient's autonomy and approves of his or her right to exercise *self-determination.* Autonomous individuals have control of their own lives and independently make their choices and decisions. This does not mean that providers are not supposed to advise their patients or recommend certain choices to them. It only entails that providers should not ignore the wishes and preferences of their patients and should avoid attempting to strongly influence patients' decisions after sufficiently educating them about the probable outcomes of each choice. As a result, the provider in this model is not an authority, but a *partner,* in the process of deciding what is best for the patient. It does not follow, however, that the provider in the autonomy-enhancing model has a passive role. To the contrary, he or she has an active but not absolute role. Such a role limits paternalism and emphasizes participation and re-spect for patients' autonomy.

EXCEPTIONS TO THE RULE

A challenging question arises at this point. Can there be exceptions to the rule that informed consent must be obtained before treating a patient? What if the patient is not mentally competent and cannot make the best choice for himself or herself? What if the patient's condition was so critical that any time spent in obtaining informed consent would be at the ex-pense of his or her life? The answer is that, like any known rule, the informed-consent rule has a few but important exceptions.

If the patient is mentally or psychologically compromised, or is expe-riencing a severe physical illness that diminishes his or her judgment, he or she cannot produce a truly informed consent. In that case, a legal repre-sentative, or **surrogate,** should be involved and should participate with the provider in decision-making. This precaution prevents the undesir-able scenario where a provider, who knows little about the social, finan-cial, or family background of the patient, makes decisions that, despite the good intentions behind them, could disrupt the life of the patient.

But suppose that the patient was in critical condition and talking with a surrogate will result in delaying urgently needed treatment. What could be done in such a case? Obviously, the provider should act from paternal-ism here. That is, he or she must do what is best for the patient and what causes the least harm. True, the provider would be violating the patient's right to autonomy. Yet he or she would be acting in good faith to enhance the patient's right to life. So adopting paternalism in this condition is morally warranted.

There are situations, however, that are more complicated than the situations of mental incompetence and emergencies. Suppose that the patient is a competent adult woman who tells her provider that she will never accept a treatment that causes her to lose her hair, no matter what. Unfortunately, the most effective treatment for her severe and life-threatening condition is a chemotherapeutic compound that leads in most cases to hair loss. Could the provider, with the intention of helping her recover from a serious disease, lie to her by denying that such a complication is feasible? Consider a similar example. A clinician exam-ines a male patient who fears having a hereditary fatal disease because his father and two brothers died of the same condition after years of suffering from both the illness and the side effects of treatment. This patient makes it clear to his provider that if he was found to have that disease, he would refuse any medication and die in peace. But the provider realizes that although the patient has the disease that killed his family members, it is still in its early stages and is likely to be mild and more responsive to therapy. If the clinician tells the patient the full truth, he would not accept any treatment, given his present state of mind. Could the clinician deceive this patient by telling him that his condition is superficially similar but fundamentally different from his father's and brothers' disease?

The latter questions are not easy to answer. In cases like that, the judgment of the provider should be individualized and adapted to the surrounding circumstances. If the woman who fears hair loss more than dying of a malignant disease seems an unreasonable person to the provider, the provider could stress the point that hair loss is a statistical finding and that she may be among the lucky people who escape this adverse reaction. If that attempt fails, the provider could refer the patient to a counselor. The assumption here is that she is likely to change her attitude in light of professional counseling before the drug causes hair loss. A counselor may enable her to think more rationally about her life and health. Yet if counseling fails and she refuses to continue treatment, the provider has to withhold the drug and offer an alternative, even if it is a less effective drug. But if she seems reasonable to the provider in her first visit, he could try a long session of education about the pros and cons of treatment versus preserving hair, then get an informed consent. There is no simple answer for such a situation, and the possibility of adopting a paternalist attitude remains a viable, last resort.

The case of the male patient who refuses treatment for a disease that killed his brothers and father can be handled on similar lines. Counseling, whether by the provider or a psychologist, could help. Any information withheld to avoid the consequences of psychological trauma should be fully disclosed upon the patient's recovery from the initial psychological trauma. Otherwise, providers should not enforce treatment on competent patients who are not in life-threatening situations. At the same time, refusal to give informed consent should not be considered the end of discussion unless the patient was educated in depth about his or her condition. In other words, refusal of consent must be an informed refusal, and this is the provider's responsibility. Patients can refuse treatment but they are entitled to know what would happen to them if they reject treatment and what they could gain if they accept treatment.

There are patients who prefer not to be informed. They find it upsetting to know about their condition in detail and think that they could deal better with it if they let the clinician make all decisions. In other words, they opt for the harm-avoidance/paternalism context. Should these patients be forced to know about their condition and the recommended treatment? This is a tricky question. To start with, people have the right to determine what is going to be done to their health. This is simply entailed by the right to autonomy. Yet people are entitled to *waive* their rights. You may have the legal right to inherit your parents' wealth but choose to waive it so that your younger disabled sister can get it and use it for her basic needs. The court cannot reject your waiver as long as it was made voluntarily. The same principle applies to waiving the right to be informed. In that case, the provider should accept the waiver and begin treatment.

Another difficult question needs to be addressed. Suppose that you are treating a child whose parents do not believe in pharmacological therapy because their religion recommends prayer as the only valid method of healing. Would you let the young daughter suffer major problems because of failure to obtain consent from her parents? Remember that the right to autonomy is purely individual. That is, each person has the right to determine his or her life, but not anyone else's life. Remember also that parents do not own their children. They are merely entitled to make decisions that enhance their well being. A parent, for example, cannot choose to let a child die when it is possible to save the life. Autonomy does not allow the parent to act on behalf of the child if the action does not promote the child's well being. True, this parent is entitled to commit suicide. This is a matter of autonomy and personal choice. But the parent is not entitled to kill a child, because autonomy does not extend to children or other persons. Therefore, a provider facing such a problem should act in the best interest of the child and should seek legal help to stop the parents from harming their child. In such situations, the provider would be acting from benevolence (beneficence and nonmaleficence).

In dentistry, there are situations where parents neglect to give care to their children because they believe primary teeth are not important and that these teeth will be replaced. Oral health care providers, in most cases, need to educate the parents about the role of primary teeth. Failing to seek the necessary treatment for their children, despite education by the dental hygienist, is neglect. In fact, neglect could be reported to social services as a form of child abuse (see Chapter 6 "Social Issues").

▬ THE IDEAL CONTEXT

As already seen, full disclosure to the patient about his or her condition and providing helpful explanations of available treatment choices are essential for obtaining informed consent. Table 3–1 lists criteria necessary for informed consent. Also, as discussed, avoiding paternalism and allowing the patient to make reasonable choices is crucial. But there are other precautions that can significantly help attaining the goal of effectively informing patients so that they can submit well-founded consent. For example, the following information must be given to the patient or to the surrogate or legal guardian in plain, understandable language:

- The diagnosis, or description of the problem.
- The nature and predicted course of the condition, both with and without treatment. The prognosis of untreated conditions and the possible cost of nontreatment, if known, should also be explained.
- Whether there is a need for certain procedures.
- Finally, the advantages, disadvantages, potential risks, cost, and long-term effects of all treatment alternatives, as well as the estimated time for treatment and the expected effect on the patient's job performance during treatment.

These considerations are relevant to daily practice of dentistry and dental hygiene. For example, in deciding to use an esthetic material or an

Table 3–1 Criteria for Informed Consent

Competency of patient confirmed

Understandable language used

Diagnosis documented

Need for treatment clarified

Prognosis explained

Alternative treatments stated
  advantages/benefits
  disadvantages/risks/side-effects

Cost specified

Length of treatment discussed

Provider of treatment specified

amalgam, the patient would have to know the advantage and disadvantage of each, such as the effect on the color of teeth or general appearance. A patient who smokes heavily and will need esthetic restorations replaced several times, due to staining, may make a decision that differs from a nonsmoker's decision. Full disclosure will help them both to decide. Similarly, patients may opt for a treatment that an insurance policy covers, although such a treatment may seem less effective to the hygienist.

DeVore (1997) suggests that informed consent ought also to include informing the patient about who will be performing the procedure (p. 60). In dentistry there is a cross-utilization of personnel for procedures. Unfortunately, patients are sometimes left unaware of the educational background, licensure status, and other qualifications of the provider who is performing a procedure. It is common that the dental hygienist, preceptor dental hygienist, certified dental assistant, and office-trained personnel may perform some of the same procedures. They have different education and may at times be performing procedures contrary to the State Dental Practice Act. For example, compare your education as a dental hygienist to the education of a dental assistant: with four hours of education, the dental assistant can legally apply pit and fissure sealants; with six hours of education, he or she can polish teeth; and with no educational requirement, the dental assistant can give fluoride treatments. Most patients rely on dentists' judgment and trust that dentists will not delegate procedures to employees who are not capable of performing them or legally allowed to perform them. But this constitutes consent based on trust, not an informed consent. Consequently, patients in dental settings should be informed about the qualifications of personnel regarding a specific procedure and should be allowed to choose who is to treat them. Informed consent means consenting to treatment. It also should mean consenting to who will be providing the treatment, although this is not always the case. In this context, it would be appropriate to remind dental hygienists that they can facilitate informed consent while enhancing the profession of dental hygiene by informing patients about the educational standards of the dental hygiene profession.

DISCLOSURE IN THE OFFICE: PRACTICAL HINTS

In practice, the estimated time needed for completing treatment should be disclosed. Patients need to know how long a treatment will take: the number of visits and the length of each visit. This helps the patient in scheduling time, dealing with insurance requirements, and arranging a payment plan. For example, patients who need extensive debridement will schedule several appointments over a relatively extended time with the hygienist. It is the dental hygienist's responsibility to inform the patient what the debridement procedure entails in terms of time and cost, even if the dentist or other authorized personnel, such as an office manager, has already given the patient a general idea. Adjunct procedures, such as oral irrigation, that are considered part of the consented treatment and any anticipated problems or discomfort after treatment should also be discussed with the patient before initiation of treatment by the dental hygienist. For treatment that is estimated to take over a year, the consent should be written.

Dental hygienists should be aware that cost is an important component of informed consent. Patients need to know the cost of treatment before they can commit to a lengthy treatment or confirm coverage with their insurers. Comparing costs of alternative treatments can help patients make a choice between them. For example, a patient may prefer an amalgam over an esthetic restoration on the basis of cost. Similarly, cost may influence the decision of the patient to choose between having a crown or a large restoration.

For financial reasons, patients covered by insurance companies or health care management organizations need to know what procedures are covered by their plans. If dentists or dental hygienists recommend procedures or intervals that are not covered, patients should be helped to know the estimated out-of-pocket cost. For example, a health care plan may cover only one prophylaxis per year; however, the dental hygienist may recommend that a more frequent debridement schedule is required for a specific periodontal condition. The patient should know the cost that is not covered by the health care plan before making a commitment. This situation is frequently encountered while practicing dental hygiene, and the prospective hygienist should be prepared to handle it. Likewise, if the dentist recommends an esthetic restoration while the health care plan covers only amalgam, the patient should be aware of the difference in cost before agreeing to the recommended form of treatment.

Communication is the core of informed consent. An open and trusting relationship needs to be developed between the patient and the health care provider. Trust cannot develop without full disclosure of all information. It is important for the hygienist to realize that disclosure may need to be repeated because many patients forget or pay insufficient attention at times. Also, patients should be allowed enough time to adapt the cost to their financial situation. No patient should be made to feel that he or she must agree "right now." Patients should be given time to think over their decisions, as quick decisions may not be rational decisions (i.e., an atmosphere of unnecessary urgency may impair judgment).

Prospective hygienists have to recognize that some patients cannot understand technical or scientific language. Using medical terminology or giving a patient literature to read is not always appropriate. Frequently, published information is "user friendly" only for well-educated patients. The information required for obtaining consent has to be given in a way that is comprehended by the patient, and plain language is always preferable. Furthermore, for informed consent to be complete, the patient should be encouraged to ask questions, and the practitioner must ensure that the patient understands every aspect of his or her treatment plan. Occasionally, it may be appropriate to ask a patient to reiterate the conveyed information to verify complete understanding of recommended treatments. In summary, communication while obtaining informed consent should be based on mutual trust, which requires full disclosure, repetition, listening to the patient's preferences, and allowing time for decision making.

Just as patients have a right to consent to treatment, they also have the right to refuse. For example, patients have the right to refuse treatment based on religious beliefs. Although these may not seem the decisions of "rational" individuals, health care providers must respect these decisions as long as they are not made on behalf of children or incompetent relatives. Christian Scientists, for instance, utilize individuals who are recognized as healers by prayer (as opposed to conventional medical treatment) and these individuals are recognized as practitioners and reimbursed for their services through various insurance companies (Dsautels, Batin, & May, 1999, p. 11). Dental hygienists are expected to respect such beliefs and practices. However, when the patient refuses the recommended treatment, the hygienist must document this in writing (Pollack & Marinelli, 1998). If the hygienist thinks that rejecting conventional treatment may lead to deleterious effects on the patient's health, she or he should carefully inform the patient of such effects. Documenting the refusal of the patient and the information given to him is equivalent to what is called *informed refusal form,* which has legal importance. As with other documentation, the patient's refusal and the advice given to him should be dated and signed by health care provider, patient, and witness. A copy of this completed form should be given to the patient (Darby & Walsh, 1995, p. 1087). In addition, there should be documentation as to why the patient is refusing treatment. If the health care provider feels that he or she can no longer render any services to the patient based on the refusal to adhere to recommended treatment, then the patient needs to be informed of this in writing.

INFORMED CONSENT AND RESEARCH

Most of the time, dental research is conducted in an institutional facility. As a dental hygienist who is employed outside of private practice, you may be involved in research with hospitals, public health departments, research centers, or other nontraditional dental hygiene practice locations. In addition, manufacturing companies may ask practicing dental hygienist to evaluate new materials on the market. Like all kinds of medical and health research, dental research may involve human subjects. This is required for advancing dental science and knowledge. But the rights of human subjects participating in research should be respected, including the right to full disclosure about the involved procedures. This is why informed consent is a necessary component of research. Research on human subjects has to be approved by an ethics or human-subjects committee (or internal review board) of the institution or agency that is sponsoring or conducting the research. Approving research on human subjects is conditional upon ascertaining that the research project is needed and has scientific value, and that it includes no risky procedures. In some cases, however, procedures involving a reasonable degree of risk may be allowed if it is believed that the potential benefit of such procedure outweighs its risk. A written consent form has to be signed by the participants. This form has to be dated and witnessed, and should include all the components of informed consent for nonresearch procedures. For example, the nature of the study, procedures used, risks, benefits, and length of time should be specified. Participants are also given verbal information regarding the study.

Participants sign a consent form indicating that they have volunteered for the study and that they were not coerced into participating or prohibited from withdrawing from the study at any time. In addition, a contact person, such as the principal investigator, along with contact information should be clearly indicated on the form. This ensures that a participant suffering from adverse effects of an experimental procedure can be promptly helped.

Some participants in research are paid for their time and effort. Details of payment as well as other material benefits should also be outlined. It is appropriate at this point to recall Kant's principle of treating persons as ends rather than as means (see Chapter 1, "Introduction to Moral Philosophy and Moral Reasoning"). This principle should be followed when researchers decide to experiment on human beings.

DISCLOSURE BY INFECTED HEALTH CARE PROVIDERS

As discussed earlier, informed consent requires that patients be informed of all possible risks before agreeing to treatment. Does that also mean that health care providers infected with blood-borne viruses such as hepatitis B or HIV should inform their patients? It is possible that practitioners who do not adhere to strict precaution measures infect their patients. In fact, the only documentation of a patient obtaining HIV from a health care practitioner has been in dentistry, although it was not possible to determine how the virus was transferred (Centers for Disease Control, 1990, 1998; Kessler, Brick, Pottage, & Benson, 1992, p. 666). In the early 1990s, the Centers for Disease Control (CDC), the American Medical Association (AMA) and the American Dental Association (ADA) issued recommendations for health care providers who were HIV-infected. These interim recommendations stated that HIV-positive providers who perform invasive procedures should stop practicing or inform their patients of their status. These guidelines relied on the principle of nonmaleficence to protect patients from a provider who could potentially harm them.

Later, the recommendations were revised and the new guidelines stated that health care providers *do not need* to be tested for HIV and they *do not need* to disclose their HIV status to their patients. But infected providers are required to consult with review panels so that the necessary precautions in each case can be determined. This modification was based partly on the right of infected providers to privacy and confidentiality, and partly on the rarity of reported cases of HIV transmission from providers to patients. For some individuals, this modification left some questions about safety of patients unanswered and raised ethical dilemmas for health care providers, although it included important guidelines.

The newly proposed guidelines include adherence to universal precautions and identification of exposure-prone invasive procedures, which are to be handled with utmost caution. It was decided that providers should know their HIV status (although they are not required to disclose it) and abstain from performing exposure-prone invasive procedures on patients without discussing the matter with review panels (Centers for Disease Control, 1991; Glasntz, Marine & Annas, 1992, p. 48). Thus the responsibility for protecting patients was assigned to members of health care professions and mandatory testing for health care workers was considered unnecessary. Obviously, if these precautions are strictly followed, the probability of patients being infected by HIV-positive practitioners who know that they are seropositive would be very low. However, a provider who is unaware of his or her HIV status may accidentally infect a patient while performing an invasive procedure. It is likely that the guidelines will be further modified if more cases of HIV transmission from clinicians to patients are discovered.

The ethical question here is, which right takes precedence: the patient's right to safety or the provider's right to privacy? Proponents of patients' rights point to the right to safety of the patient and insist that it is the provider's duty to disclose his or her HIV status. Advocates of privacy argue that the likelihood of infection is so low that disclosure is unnecessary. Perhaps the CDC recommendations strike a balance between both points of view, and time will show how adequate these recommendations are.

It is very important to realize that dental and dental hygiene procedures are exposure-prone because they are invasive due to the use of needles (either for injections or sutures) and sharp instruments in highly confined areas with poor visibility. Therefore, it is imperative that clinical dental hygienists be constantly aware of their own HIV status. A hygienist who turns positive is required to accept the judgment of a review panel or to disclose her or his status to patients. This is not only a legal issue. It is also, and primarily, an ethical one. The only other option for such a hygienist is to withdraw from clinical practice.

PATIENTS' BILL OF RIGHTS

Patients are guaranteed information regarding their care not only through informed consent but also through the **patients' bill of rights.** This bill typically outlines what the patient can expect as a partner in his or her own health care. The wording of the bill may vary from one facility to another, but the fundamental rights are usually stated everywhere. The bill includes the patients' right to be informed and to accept or refuse treatment or participation in research. Also, the bill assures patients that they are entitled to know who is treating them, which external agencies are affiliated with the facility providing care, and the rules regulating charges and payments. The bill also endorses the patients' right to know of any alternatives to the proposed treatment. Private dental offices may or may not have their own patients' bill of rights (see Table 3–2). The patients' bill of rights is usually displayed in visible places such as the reception areas of a healthcare facility but copies may also be distributed with other forms that the patient has access to, such as informed consent or "new patient introductory forms" (Dietz, 2000, p. 117). However, many clinics, hospitals, and other dental treatment centers display this bill as a part of their

Table 3–2   A Concise Version of Patients' Bill of Rights for Dental
Hygiene Practice

We strive to consider *patients as partners* in their oral health care and in meeting their oral health care needs. As patients in our care, you can expect the following:

• You will be treated with respect, dignity, and courtesy.

• Information about your health will be confidential and privacy will be maintained.

• You will be informed of length of appointments and fees before scheduling services. Appointments will be kept and a reasonable fee will be charged. You will be made aware of insurance and payment arrangements.

• You will be kept informed of your dental and dental hygiene needs, progress of treatment, and any change in treatment conditions.

• You will be encouraged to seek alternative treatment, referrals, and second opinions when necessary.

• You will have access to your dental and dental hygiene records.

• You will have the right to refuse treatment.

Note: Adapted from Dietz, 2000, p. 118.

policy. For example, a dental clinic in a hospital may display the patients' bill of rights created by the American Hospital Association.

The United States Congress proposed the Patients' Bill of Rights Act of 1999 to help patients, as consumers, make decisions regarding health services and benefits. This legislation will help consumers obtain health coverage and increase the country's health care systems, quality of health, and research. (Patients Bill of Rights Act, 1999). This Act seeks to protect patients, as consumers, by expanding disclosure requirements, grievances, appeals, reviews, and genetic nondiscrimination provisions found in health care plans. Ideally, the Act will promote better access to care and quality of care as patients are allowed to question treatment decisions, such as emergency room visits and referrals to specialists, determined by their health care plans and primary care providers.

SUMMARY

Informed consent consists of two components: information for the patient and consent by the patient. The patient must be informed of the recommended treatment, its risks, and alternative treatments. Exceptions to informed consent occur in situations of emergencies and mental incompetence. Patients are also entitled to refuse treatment after being informed about its importance and about the consequences of refusal. Surrogate decision makers (i.e., parents or legal guardians) must be informed when patients cannot make decisions for themselves (e.g., patients in coma or children) and are supposed to consider the best interest of the patients. Patients may also waiver the right to informed consent; that is, they may not want to be involved in decisions regarding treatment. Applying the therapeutic principle, health care providers can also withhold information from patients if it is in the interest of the patients not to be told. There is controversy regarding the right of patients to know whether their health care providers are infected with HIV or similar infectious illnesses, but reasonable guidelines have been issued by the CDC to protect patients without violating the privacy of providers. The patients' bill of rights provides additional assurances for patients about their entitlement to know about and accept or reject a recommended treatment.

SELF-TEST

1. Informed consent consists of the health care provider giving _____ and the patient giving _____.
   a) information, approval
   b) consent, information
   c) treatment, approval
   d) services, payment
2. A patient can refuse treatment that he or she needs if all the following criteria are met *unless* the patient
   a) is not a minor.
   b) has a mental condition that impairs judgment.
   c) was informed of the prognosis in absence of treatment.
   d) none of the above.
3. Name the criteria for informed consent.
4. Informed consent allows the patient to be a partner in treatment.
   a) True
   b) False
5. Informed consent includes the patient's right to refuse treatment.
   a) True
   b) False

6. Informed consent upholds the ethical principle of
    a) autonomy.
    b) parentalism.
    c) confidentiality.
    d) documentation.
7. Informed consent involves telling the patient
    a) the diagnosis.
    b) the treatment alternatives.
    c) the risks involved for each treatment.
    d) all the above.

ACTIVITIES

1. Divide into pairs. Role play the following activities:
    a) Ask for *informed consent* from a patient for dental hygiene periodontal therapy. This patient has never had debridement or prophylaxis treatment, but has had limited restorative treatment. The patient comes from a background where one visited the dentist only if one was in pain. There is heavy calculus and generalized pockets of 4 to 6mm.
    b) Ask for *informed consent* from a parent for a minor to receive x-rays, pit and fissure sealants, and fluoride treatment in addition to the scheduled examination and prophylaxis.
    c) Ask for *informed consent* from a female patient of childbearing age for local anesthesia.
    d) Ask for *informed consent* from a 55 year-old male patient for nitrous oxide-oxygen sedation.
2. Read the *patients' bill of rights* posted in your dental hygiene program. Are there any items that you would like to add?
3. Give examples or develop scenarios where it would be appropriate for the dental hygienist to apply the principle of paternalism through nondisclosure.

CASE STUDY

Contributed by Debi Gerger, RDH, BS, MPH Program/Clinic Coordinator, San Joaquin Valley College, Rancho Cucamonga CA.

Scenario: As a registered dental hygienist, you perform intraoral and extraoral soft tissue examination on all patients at the recall visits. Today, your first patient is someone you have been treating for three years. In the past you noted a white lesion on her left buccal mucosa that has become larger at each recall. Today, it appears to have become indurated and is white with a red border. Because you do not want to alarm your patient, you do not say anything until the dentist comes to do the exam. The patient states that she bit her cheek a couple of days ago. The dentist evaluates the lesion, but does not see any reason for concern. The dentist recommends reevaluation of the area at the next recall visit. Recognize that the patient is not aware of the terms that you and the dentist are using. The patient does understand that the dentist is not concerned.

Discussion: Consider why the dentist is choosing to ignore the lesion. Was the patient convincing that the lesion was just a bite? Is the dentist ill informed about diagnosing lesions? Does the dentist feel uncomfortable informing patients about potential cancer? Did the hygienist not inform the dentist of the past history of the lesions? Is it noted in the patient's chart? Has she been informed of it previously?

As the chapter discusses, informed consent involves telling the patient of all potential causes of the lesion and then allowing time for the patient to ask questions. Although some of the information that we must deliver may not be pleasant, we still have an obligation to inform the patient. We must remember to be careful in regards to diagnosing, though. In most states dental hygienists can record and inform patients of their assessment findings, but are not allowed to diagnose. In this case, like most, the patient would like to believe that there is nothing wrong. What will you do?

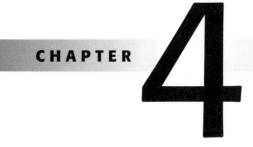

Decision Making

OBJECTIVES

Upon reading the material in this chapter, you will be able to

1. Define the term *ethical dilemma*.
2. List the steps involved in ethical decision making.
3. Solve ethical dilemmas using a decision making process.
4. Determine core values and principles used to solve an ethical dilemma.
5. Discuss the role of laws in determining alternatives for solving an ethical dilemma.

INTRODUCTION

Throughout our lives we are faced with the necessity of **decision making.** Decision making is a process utilizing critical-thinking skills to arrive at a judgment or conclusion. Before you entered dental hygiene, you made the decision to continue your education. Then you decided where to enroll. Later, as a student, you may have had to make the decision to work on weekends to support yourself. After graduation, you will make many other decisions. Life is full of situations that require decisions, and some decisions are difficult to make.

Dental hygienists make decisions daily. In the treatment of patients, dental hygienists constantly are utilizing critical-thinking skills. For example, they use decision making in selecting the type of fluoride to use for a patient with ceramic crowns. Although the majority of dental hygienists work under the supervision of dentists, dental hygienists are responsible for the dental hygiene diagnosis and dental hygiene treatment plans. As members of a profession, dental hygienists have autonomy in these decisions and should provide treatment that meets the acceptable *standard of care* for all dental hygiene procedures. At times, however, the decisions may not be easy. For instance, the dentist's line of treatment and referral (or lack of referral) may conflict with the treatment plan designed by the dental hygienist. In this situation, the dental hygienist may choose to follow the suggestions of the dentist or ignore them and risk losing her or his job.

Similarly, the dental hygienist's treatment plan may conflict with the patient's insurance company's coverage plan, which may not cover the preferred treatment. In that case, the dental hygienist may decide to modify the plan to agree with the insurance policy or to let the patient decide whether to pay the extra cost. In the former example, there was a conflict between two interpretations of the patient's best interest: one offered by the dentist and the other by the hygienist. But the conflict was technical or practical. In the latter example, the conflict arose between the administrative policy of the insurance company and the treatment plan. Yet it was also a practical conflict because it concerned financial issues without endangering the patient's oral health.

But not all the conflicts that dental hygienist confront are technical or practical. They also meet with moral (ethical) conflicts. Suppose that the dental hygienist finds that his or her patient needs referral to a periodontist for an effective treatment, but the dentist does not like to refer patients whenever he or she could perform a useful but less effective treatment at the office. This hypothetical dentist may have reasons for withholding referrals. He or she may be interested in maximizing income or in practicing a technique that was recently learned. The dentist may be concerned that many referred patients lose their tie with the office and never come back. The situation here is not merely practical. It has a moral dimension. The basic issue is not the patient's best interest but the dentist's self-interest. The patient is not treated as an end in himself or herself, but as means.

Consider another example. Suppose that a patient has an old restoration that needs replacement, but the policy of the office is to prophylactically replace all old restorations, regardless of their condition. The assumption here is that old restorations will eventually deteriorate, no matter what. Should the dental hygienist volunteer to tell the patient that the benefit from replacing all old restorations at present is questionable and that the patient should make it clear that he or she wants only defective restorations replaced? This hygienist faces two incompatible choices: to comply with the policy of the office or to give priority to the best interest of patients. This situation also has a moral aspect.

ETHICAL DILEMMA

A **dilemma** is a situation necessitating a choice between two equal, especially undesirable, alternatives. For example, if a person has to choose either to buy a new car and be in debt for several years or to keep an old car and spend a lot of money on mechanical repairs, he or she is confronting a dilemma. An **ethical dilemma** may be defined as a conflict between moral obligations that are difficult to reconcile (Honderich, 1995, p. 201). An example of a person facing an ethical dilemma is a single mother whose elderly and disabled parents need her care, but who cannot care for them and her children without giving up her full-time job. At the same time, she cannot quit her job before her children finish their education and are able to support themselves. This person, obviously, is not in a position to fulfill the obligations imposed on her in an adequate way. The dilemma she is facing is not practical, but ethical, because it involves the well-being of other persons and her duties towards them.

Ethical dilemmas are challenges that require moral reasoning. Moral reasoning, in turn, needs to be guided by ethical principles. In this example, the single mother could use the utilitarian and beneficence principles to choose the arrangement that does the least harm to each involved party.

Dental hygienists may confront similar ethical dilemmas. There will always be situations that require satisfying multiple parties. The best interest of the patient is not always compatible with the interests of insurance companies, hospitals, dentists, or other care providers. The dental hygienist must take into consideration the conflicting interests of all parties. He or she may find that the amount of work needed for a nursing-institution patient cannot be done without disrupting the budget of that institution. The scarcity of these funds leaves the dental hygienist in a dilemma.

Dental hygienists should be prepared to deal with ethical dilemmas in efficient ways. Like the single mother in the previous example, the dental hygienist needs ethical principles to resolve dilemmas.

The core values (discussed in Chapter 2, "Ethical Principles and Core Values") found in the Code of Ethics of the ADHA may be a good starting point in solving ethical dilemmas. They provide dental hygienists with general strategies of action that, if followed, are likely to lead to the most acceptable results. For instance, they inform the dental hygienist of the importance of preserving societal trust in all situations. Consequently, when the best interest of the patient conflicts with the best interest of the public, the hygienist would have to find a compromise that furthers the patient's interests without jeopardizing public trust. For instance, it may be in the best interest of some patients to use cosmetically appealing materials (such as ceramic inlays). But the public may not accept paying higher insurance premiums or paying out of pocket to cover the cost of such materials. In that case, the dental hygienist should balance the preferences of the patient with those of society. Otherwise, dental hygienists may lose the trust of the public.

However, the Code of Ethics of the ADHA does not provide guidelines for every situation. In fact, all codes of ethics are intended to reinforce and complement, rather than to replace, the reasoning capability of professionals. As a dental hygienist, you will need to utilize other means of problem solving when you face a dilemma. In addition to the code of ethics, you may draw on reasoning skills that you acquired throughout your life by socialization, previous experience, learning from role models, formal ethical education, and even *gut feeling* (or intuition). Dental hygienists facing ethical dilemmas utilize, in addition to the principles stressed by their code of ethics, advice from peers, legal advice, and their personal experiences. They also consider legal and administrative consequences while making decisions regarding ethical problems. However, the way an ethical dilemma is solved should in the end conform to the moral principles and core values discussed in previous chapters.

Think about the following case scenario. A woman has been receiving *routine* care since childhood. She has now moved from her hometown and comes to your office as a new patient for her 6-month dental hygiene prophylaxis. You initiate your appointment with a review of her medical history, radiographs, probing, and other assessment measures. This patient has generalized bleeding and localized pockets. You find heavy subgingival calculus, especially in the interproximal posterior regions. Your patient needs to return for another appointment. She questions why she needs to return and why you did a lot of "extras" before you started treatment with the ultrasonic scaler. She states that in the previous office, her appointments always were completed within one hour and the dental hygienist always complimented her on how well she took care of her teeth.

This poses an ethical dilemma. Would you tell the patient that she had previously been given poor treatment that was not current with standard of care? Or, do you continue to treat her in the manner she is accustomed to and compromise your treatment? The first choice may lead to a loss of societal trust in dental hygiene. The public expects dental hygienists to provide high quality of care. Also, pointing to the faults of colleagues undermines societal trust. At the same time, the second choice implies giving substandard care to the patient. If you were the dental hygienist, how would you resolve this dilemma?

Consider a patient who is also a mother. She asks you to write an absentee form stating that she needs another appointment so that she can take a sick day from work to be with her child for a school recital. You know that it is morally wrong to lie, yet you appreciate how important it is to both mother and child that she attend the recital. Should you lie for the parent and arrange for the requested absence form? How would this lie be perceived? Should you suggest that the mother explain to her child how difficult it is to leave work and hope that the child will understand and accept the situation? What is your position on this situation?

DEVELOPING THE ABILITY TO SOLVE ETHICAL PROBLEMS

It is important to realize that there are several factors that influence our decision making in solving ethical dilemmas. We do not acquire the ability to solve ethical problems and make ethically relevant decisions overnight. Rather, it is a gradual and lengthy process that begins even before reading about morality, taking a course in ethics, or studying the ADHA Code of Ethics. You may recall that you began to think about "good" and "bad" actions in your early childhood. You may also remember how parents and teachers tried to guide your reasoning about what is good or bad by examples and anecdote or by simply giving you firm instructions. The moral conscience has its roots in early life and is influenced by cultural elements. Modern social scientists have proposed theories to explain this process. Among these theories is Kohlberg's model of moral development, which gained remarkable popularity among students of ethics. It is useful to be acquainted with that model because it highlights the gradually evolving process that leads to acquiring the ability to make ethical decisions.

Lawrence Kohlberg (1967) suggested that there are three levels and six hierarchy stages to moral development (see Table 4–1.) Each level has two stages, and each step must be reached before progressing to the next step.

Table 4–1 Levels and Stages in Moral Development

Level I	*Preconventional Level:* Moral values resides in external quasi-physical happenings, in bad acts, or in quasi-physical needs rather than in persons and standards.
	Stage 1: Orientation to punishment, obedience, and physical and material power. Rules are obeyed to avoid punishment.
	Stage 2: Naïve instrumental hedonistic orientation. The child conforms to obtain rewards.
Level II	*Conventional Level:* Moral values reside in performing good or right roles, in maintaining the conventional order and the expectations of others.
	Stage 3: "Good boy" orientation designed to win approval and maintain expectations of one's immediate group. The child conforms to avoid disapproval. One earns approval by being "nice."
	Stage 4: Orientation to authority, law, and duty to maintain a fixed order, whether social or religious. Right behavior consists of doing one's duty and abiding by the social order.
Level III	*Postconventional, Autonomous, or Principled Level:* Moral values reside in conformity by the self to shared or shareable standards, rights, and duties.
	Stage 5: Social contract orientation, in which duties are defined in terms of contract and the respect of others' rights. Emphasis is upon equality and mutual obligations within a democratic order. There is an awareness of relativism of personal values and the use of procedural rules in reaching consensus.
	Stage 6: The morality of individual principles of conscience that have logical comprehensiveness, universality, and consistency. These principles are not concrete (like the Ten Commandments) but general and abstract (like the Golden Rule, the categorical imperative).

Note. From *Moral development: Text and readings,* A. G. Oldenquist, 1978, Boston: Houghton Mifflin; and *Theories of moral development,* J. M. Rich and J. L. DeVitis, 1985, Springfield, IL: Charles C. Thomas.

The three levels are preconventional, conventional, and postconventional. The basic assumption of his theory is that as individuals pass through these stages, they progressively utilize thinking and problem solving more than fixed rules to solve ethical dilemmas. But to reach the stage of thinking rather than just following fixed rules, one needs to gain cognitive development. Cognitive development means developing knowledge of the moral values and standards of one's group or society. Having such knowledge is essential for developing the ability to make moral judgments.

Kohlberg based this theory on his study of males of different ages, different socioeconomic backgrounds, and different cultures. His findings suggest that children tend to solve problems at a simple level, which he described as Stages 1 and 2. Most adults, however, tend to operate at a more complex level, described as Stages 3 and 4. But only 20 percent of the population were able to reach a higher level of moral reasoning, and not all of them reach the final stage in that level, which Kohlberg described as Stage 6. He found that less than ten percent of the adult population operate at Stage 6. As dental hygienists, we should aspire to reach the final stage, or the most advanced level of moral reasoning in general. This will enable us to solve moral dilemmas in the most rational way. But, as Kohlberg's research shows, not many people reach this final stage. It is plausible to suggest that what is needed for reaching the most advanced stage is the study of ethics.

Among social scientists who tried to refine Kohlberg's model is James Rest. He suggested that developing cognitive dimensions to moral reasoning requires attaining other abilities. Among these abilities are having moral sensitivity, moral motivation, and moral character (Rest, 1986). While Kohlberg stressed cultural and societal influences, Rest emphasized the importance of education and personal experience. He pointed out that age and education had an effect on moral thinking; the older and more educated individuals tended to behave more morally.

This observation applies to dental hygiene students. In an important study, dental hygiene students who had more formal education were found to have more advanced moral reasoning ability than those who had less formal education (Newell, Young, & Yamoor, 1985). Bebeau, Rest, and Yamoor (1985) reported similar results with dental students: Third-year dental students reasoned at a higher level than first-year dental students, and faculty reasoned at a higher level than students. These studies support the notion that dental hygienists can better serve their clients (and society in general) by attaining the highest possible level of education, which should include ethical education. The awareness of the basic principles of morality, which are discussed in the opening chapters of this book, is very important for making sound ethical decisions. It would be useful for dental hygienists to reflect on this account and adapt it to the dilemmas that they encounter in their practice. It is particularly useful to capture its emphasis on the significance of having the desire and motivation to act morally in all situations.

STEPS OF DECISION MAKING

Decision making, as already defined, is a process that utilizes critical thinking to make a judgment or to reach a conclusion. Critical thinking is reasoning in an objective, organized, and logical manner. In clinical dental hygiene practice, we often use critical thinking to formulate a dental hygiene care plan based on the treatment categories: assessment, dental hygiene diagnosis, planning, implementation (Mueller-Joseph & Petersen, 1995, p. 2; Wilkins, 1999, p. 321). Similarly, decision making in ethical contexts requires critical thinking. Like practical problems, an ethical problem or dilemma cannot be solved in a subjective or arbitrary manner. Good reasoning is our best tool for solving problems, whether they are clinical, scientific, administrative, or ethical. This is why dealing with ethical problems proceeds on lines similar to those followed in solving clinical problems in dental hygiene practice.

To simplify the process of decision making in various situations, many authors propose models for solving dilemmas. However, most of these models involve, in some form or another, the same steps. Typically, making a decision starts with identifying the problem then proceeds to gathering the relevant facts. Having done that, the person dealing with the problem lays out the alternative solutions, evaluates them, then selects the most appropriate course of action. While acting to solve the problem, the person continues to evaluate the selected action to ensure its merits. An action that survives such evaluation is continued until the problem is resolved. These steps, which are adapted from several models, are summarized in Table 4–2.

Ethical dilemmas are usually solved in a similar way. For example, Darby and Walsh (1995) and Purtilo (1999) proposed schemes for solving ethical dilemmas that, in essence, simulate the above steps. Their schemes, however, use specific terms that match the ethical context. For instance,

Table 4–2   Steps in Decision Making

Identifying the problem	Define the problem or dilemma
Gathering the facts	Be a detective; ask questions
Listing the alternatives	Brainstorm; list pros and cons
Selecting the course of action	Justify the chosen action
Acting on the decision	Follow through on decision
Evaluating the action	Judge the results of the action

selecting the course of action is called "establishing an ethical position," and consulting theories of ethics is recommended for accomplishing this step. Purtilo recommends utilizing normative ethical theories and taking into consideration the principles stressed by deontology, utilitarianism, and other ethical positions (see discussion in Chapter 1, "Introduction to Moral Philosophy and Moral Reasoning") while selecting a course of action. Rule and Veatch (1993) recommend also considering the principles adopted by the Dental Hygiene Code of Ethics at this step.

At this point it would be useful to reformulate the steps of decision making in a way that enables the dental hygienist to solve ethical dilemmas arising in daily practice. Weinstein (1993) offers the following adaptation of the decision making steps to guide solving ethical dilemmas facing dental hygienists.

1. Gather the dental, medical, social, and all other clinically relevant facts of the case.
2. Identify all relevant values that play a role in the case and determine which values, if any, are in conflict.
3. List the options open to you to deal with the problem.
4. Choose the best solution from an ethical point of view.
5. Justify this solution.
6. Respond to possible criticism of the selected solution (p. 44).

Explaining Decision Making Steps

The steps required for decision making may be further understood in light of the following explanations.

IDENTIFYING THE PROBLEM

Before we can solve a problem, we need to know its dimensions and implications. In other words, we should be able to determine what needs to be solved. This involves analyzing the problem and finding out whether it involves any violation of ethical principles. It is crucial to clearly determine whether there is an actual ethical dilemma, just a clash of personalities, or different interpretations of the issue. So, identifying the problem includes deciding whether the problem is an ethical dilemma. This is not always obvious. Good questions to ask are: Is it a matter of the way things are "done in the office" versus lack of *standard of care* or a matter of following the Dental Practice Act versus following the Code of Ethics? Is it a conflict between self-interest and acting morally?

Gathering the Facts

There is an old axiom that says "don't assume anything." In solving an ethical dilemma it may be necessary to act as a detective, to ask the *what, when, where, why,* and *how* questions. We must also clarify assumptions and separate them from facts. Moreover, we must be aware of available sources of information about the relevant issue. In a study of dental students and how they would solve ethical dilemmas, it was found that they were not aware of certain avenues open to them. For example, in finding low quality dental care in a new patient, dental students did not think of contacting a dental review board or a dentist who had done previous dental care on a patient (Bebeau, Rest, & Yamoor, 1985). This shows the importance of understanding a profession's code of ethics, standards of care, professional liabilities, and legal regulations.

Listing the Alternatives

It is always useful to have several possible solutions for a problem. Whenever there are many alternatives, a better solution is likely to be found. Brainstorming is enhanced by listing all reasonable suggestions rather sticking to one or a few alternatives. Sometimes it is the suggestion that first appeared to be the most unlikely that eventually proves to be the best. However, we must exclude unreasonable alternatives as soon as it becomes clear that they are not going to help. Alternative solutions should take into consideration the concerns and obligations (rights and duties, wants and needs) of all those involved in a situation. An alternative that ignores the interests or duties of one party is unlikely to be a reliable solution.

Sometimes an alternative seems warranted for one situation, but not for others. This is why it is important to realize that solutions should be sensitive to the context. For example, it is generally improper to allow a dental assistant or dental hygienist to perform procedures not approved by the Dental Practice Act. If you see a dental hygienist doing a procedure that the Dental Practice Act assigns only to dentists, your list of alternatives would include advising the hygienist not to do so. But suppose that a dental assistant or hygienist is very skilled at a procedure that is supposed to be done only by a dentist. You see him or her performing this procedure in a public facility in an underserved rural area, where no dentist is available. If you think in light of the nonmaleficence and utilitarian principles, you would probably find nothing wrong with that situation. Then, you may include the choice of "turning a blind eye" to the situation among your list of alternatives. If you chose not to object to the violation of the Dental Practice Act in that particular situation, you would be making a distinction between what is administratively or legally wrong and what is morally wrong. Indeed, what is legal and administratively correct is not always morally wrong, and vice versa. However, conflicts between moral and legal judgments are likely to arise only in exceptional situations.

SELECTING THE COURSE OF ACTION
Having evaluated the alternatives, we need to select the course of action. This involves weighing the negative with the positive aspects of each possible course of action. The risks involved with each action also need to be identified. That is, we should ask the question, What could go wrong if a particular course of action is selected? At the same time, we should identify the merits of each possible course of action. Could that action be defended or justified on the grounds of moral principles and the values of the code of ethics? Such a question must be answered before endorsing a course of action. The reason actions should be scrutinized at a moral level is that moral judgments should not be arbitrary.

ACTING
The aim of considering the alternatives then assessing their advantages and disadvantages is to act in light of careful analysis of the situation. Acting becomes easy when we are sure that the selected action is justifiable. The best actions are those that survive ethical scrutiny. The consequences of such actions are often rewarding. Perhaps the least desirable consequences of morally justified actions is creating a conflict of interest. When we choose an action that runs against the preferences of superiors, there is always the risk of losing a job or friendships. Sometimes, worse consequences, such as losing reputation or status in the community, follow an action that may seem wrong to those who were not aware of all the aspects of the situation. However, we must act according to moral principles and bravely face the consequences. Fortunately, there are always principled people in every society who will defend good decisions and moral actions.

EVALUATING THE ACTION
In evaluating a selected action, a good question to ask is: If it happened again, would I make the same decision? A positive answer often implies the soundness of that action. We may also determine the effect of our decisions on the growth and development of the profession. Some good ac-

tions may initially look questionable, but eventually lead to positive change in the practice of the profession. This is why we should continue to evaluate an action until all its consequences become clear. The implications of an action for ourselves, other members of the profession, and the community as a whole should be assessed. Actions that were previously evaluated and found satisfactory should be adopted, while actions that were not well received should be revised. The dental hygienist should welcome every critique and feedback about a selected action.

SUMMARY

Throughout life, individuals are faced with both personal and professional decisions. An ethical dilemma occurs when there is a conflict between moral principles. The capability to solve ethical dilemmas is acquired from the individual's progression through levels and stages of moral development. Other factors, such as age and education, gut feeling, and personality, may also determine solutions to ethical problems. Yet the awareness of moral principles and theories crucially enhances attaining this ability. There are several models of decision making, but the majority of them include identifying the problem, gathering the facts, listing the alternatives, selecting the course of action, acting, and evaluating the action.

SELF-TEST

1. The code of ethics can be used to justify a given solution to an ethical dilemma.
    a) True
    b) False
2. An *ethical dilemma* occurs when there is a conflict in the
   _____.
    a) profession.
    b) laws.
    c) morally right thing to do.
    d) none of the above.
3. All legal actions are ethical and moral.
    a) True
    b) False

4. As one gathers the facts to solve an ethical dilemma in dental hygiene practice, a useful tool may be the state practice act.
   a) True
   b) False

5. Decision making for ethical dilemmas in dental hygiene practice involve _____.
   a) code of ethics.
   b) laws.
   c) critical thinking skills.
   d) rights and duties.
   e) all the above.

6. Nothing is needed for making ethical decisions in dental hygiene practice except the ADHA Code of Ethics.
   a) True
   b) False

ACTIVITIES

1. Investigate decision making models utilized by authors to solve ethical dilemmas presented in dental and dental hygiene publications (i.e., *Probe, Journal of Dental Hygiene, Access, RDH, Practical Hygiene,* and *Journal of the American Dental Association*). Case scenarios are often included as an ongoing section or a featured item in the professional literature.

2. Create a case scenario based on your experience as a dental hygiene student. Solve the ethical dilemma, outlining each step of the solution. Share the decision making process with a fellow student, a small group of students, or the class. What role did the ADHA Code of Ethics play in your decision making? What were the perceived obstacles to overcome for moral behavior, justice, and fairness?

3. Write a one-page reaction to an ethical problem or issue discussed in either of the following articles:

CASE STUDY

Contributed by Debi Gerger, RDH, BS, MPH, Program/Clinic Coordinator, San Joaquin Valley College, Rancho Cucamonga, CA.

Scenario: You have been a practicing dental hygienist in general offices for three years. Recently, you have joined a periodontal office. The dentists in the practice have a great reputation; many of the dentists you worked for referred patients to this office. On your first day of work, the first patient is scheduled for root planing, which goes very well. Your second patient is scheduled for a periodontal maintenance. The patient has been seen regularly in this practice for two years and has 4mm to 8mm pocket probing depths. After seating the patient, you evaluate the medical history to discover that the patient has marked, on numerous occasions, that he has a heart murmur. As you question him further, he gets very upset with you because the other hygienist never asked him any of these questions, and he has never had any problems. You dismiss yourself to discuss this with the dentist. The dentist is in the middle of a surgery and quickly directs you *not* to give the patient antibiotics and to continue with the prophylaxis. The dentist has refused to premedicate the patient when you know it should be done.

In analyzing this case, consider which of the ethical principles are involved. Recognize that this case involves the dental hygienist, the dentist, and the patient.

Discussion: One of the first concerns should be why the dentist does not want to reschedule the patient after a medical consultation is completed. Is the dentist only concerned with completing the patient today? Does the dentist not know the current recommendations regarding heart conditions? Is the dentist concerned about losing the fee for the procedure?

Many of the ethical principles discussed in this chapter can be applied to this case study. The principle of *beneficence* means to do good. We must deliver the best care possible to our patients. The principle of *nonmaleficence* is similar in that it means to do no harm. We are not to knowingly place patients at risk. In this case, the patient may have been at risk for a bacteremia. The principle of *trust* can also be applied. The public trusts our profession to provide skilled and competent care. Even though this patient was upset, he still has a trust that we will not harm him.

There are a number of ways to handle this situation, some ethical and some unethical. List all of your options in this case. Which would you choose, and why?

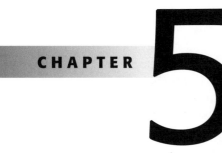

Jurisprudence

Upon reading the material in this chapter, you will be able to

1. Compare the concepts of civil law with criminal law, utilizing examples found in dental hygiene practice.
2. List the types and circumstances of *supervision* (or absence of supervision) found in the Dental Practice Act of the state in which you reside or attend school.
3. State the conditions necessary for a contract between a patient and a dental hygienist with regards to dental hygiene services.
4. Define and distinguish between the following terms:
   intentional tort and *unintentional* tort,
   malpractice and *negligence,*
   libel and *slander,*
   assault and *battery,*
   implied contract and *expressed* contract.
5. Discuss the *rights* of patients protected by law and *duties* of providers regulated by law from both *ethical* and *legal* perspectives.

INTRODUCTION

The previous chapters have discussed the role of ethics in dental hygiene practice; this chapter will discuss the role of **jurisprudence.** Jurisprudence is the science or philosophy of law (Hanks, 1986, p. 829), which may also include the establishment, regulation, and enforcement of legislation. **Statutory law** is enacted by legislation through United States Congress, state legislature, or local legislative bodies (Miller & Hutton, 2000, p. 7). The two types of statutory law are **criminal law** and **civil law.** Criminal law involves crimes against society, with the government initiating legal action, and civil law involves crimes against an individual, with the harmed individual initiating the legal action. Two subsets of civil law are tort law and contract law. Examples of laws found in dental hygiene practice are state dental practice acts, rules and regulations governing the practice of dental hygiene, discrimination laws, child abuse reporting, OSHA regulations, and insurance practices. There is a range of penalties for violation of laws, which can include an administrative warning (which amounts only to a reprimand), loss of license or suspension of license, monetary or community service fines, mandatory education (either professional continuing education or social education), and prison sentence. **Common law,** or **case law,** is formulated by judges or determined by court decisions; common law is issued through judgments, and *not* by the legislation. For example, according to common law, some couples may be considered legally married after a given number of years of living together. Scott (1998) states that laws related to health care legal and ethical issues, business relationships among health professions and organizations, and most American civil legal authority derives from common law (p. 7).

CRIMINAL LAW

Criminal law concerns offenses or wrongful acts against society and should protect the public's interest, whereas civil law concerns offenses or wrongful acts against an individual, including the individual's property and reputation. Additional comparisons between criminal law and civil law are found in Table 5–1. Criminal law seeks to punish the offender, while civil law seeks to compensate the victim (Davison, 2000, p. 34). Criminal law applies to everyone. For example, no matter who you are, it is wrong to kill or steal. In a criminal case, a jury must unanimously agree on a judgment, and the prosecutors, who represent society, must prove guilt beyond a reasonable doubt. If found guilty in a criminal case, an in-

Table 5–1 Comparison of Criminal Law and Civil Law

Item	Criminal Law	Civil Law
Initiator of Legal Action	Government (state, county, etc.)	Individual
Crime is Against	Society	Individual
Agreement of Jurors	Unanimous (all jurors)	51% (majority of jurors)
Payment of Damages	Life, liberty, fine	Nominal, compensatory, punitive
Guilty of Crime	Beyond a reasonable doubt	Responsible for the crime

dividual could lose life (death penalty), liberty (prison sentence), or be fined (payment either with money or community service).

Performing dental hygiene procedures without having a license is a violation of criminal law. The purpose of a license is to protect the public. For example, the state government grants licensure to drive a car. To drive a car, an individual needs to obtain a driver's license to prove that he or she is able to obey the traffic laws and drive safely. This is to protect the public. If a person disobeys the law, he or she may be penalized with a jail term or a monetary or community service fine. Likewise, a dental hygienist must obtain a license from the state to ensure that he or she can safely provide specific treatment to the public. When the student has completed a recognized educational program and passed both a national written board examination and a practical examination, a state agency will grant a license to practice. If an individual practices dental hygiene without a license or performs procedures not allowed by the state dental practice act, he or she is performing a criminal act, and this may be considered a felony (Pollak & Marinelli, 1988, p. 30). An individual can be jailed or fined, or his or her dental hygiene license may be revoked or suspended for not complying with the guidelines of the state dental practice act, which is legislated law.

Insurance fraud is another criminal act that may be committed in dental hygiene practice. A dental hygienist may be asked to postdate a treatment appointment. Many times insurance guidelines dictate that specific services may be performed only within a certain time period. For example, preventive dental hygiene treatment will only be reimbursed every six months. Suppose a male college student was seen by the dental hygienist in early April during spring break and wants to schedule the next appointment before school starts in the fall. He asks the dental hygienist to postdate the appointment so that the insurance company will pay for the treatment. Should the dental hygienist postdate the treatment to October and not September, then fraud has occurred. Likewise, predating treatment for insurance coverage is also fraud. A female college student, let us suppose, has graduated a month before her dental hygiene appointment and no longer has student health and dental insurance. If the dental hygienist stated that the treatment was done earlier to help this student avoid out of pocket payment, he or she is also committing insurance fraud. Other types of fraud (i.e., claiming that something was done when it was not done) may also occur in the dental hygiene employment environment, as in any other work or personal situation. Claiming that additional work was in the treatment plan when that work was not really done is like claiming more damage on a car then actually occurred in an accident. A dental hygienist could be considered guilty of fraud in certain situations, even though he or she may not have actually signed the insurance forms. If a dental hygienist is aware of a fraud committed by a patient or coworker and does not report it, he or she could be considered guilty by association. Again, this illegal fraudulent action would be tried in criminal court.

CIVIL LAW

Civil law affects the dental hygiene practice when the dental hygienist does a procedure or fails to perform a procedure and the patient brings legal action against the dental hygienist. For example, if the dental hygienist caused harm while giving local anesthetic, and it was illegal, according to the state dental practice act, for a dental hygienist to administer local anesthetic, then there has been harm against society and against the individual. This involves both criminal and civil laws.

There are three types of damage that an individual who is found guilty in civil court can be ordered to pay. The first type *is nominal*, or the actual cost of the damage. For example, the cost of actually having a car repaired or a tooth restored. The second type is *compensatory* and includes nominal damages plus extra cost incurred. Compensatory damages are imposed to compensate for the nonmaterial and material harm caused to an individual. These damages may include lost wages or salary, pain and suffering, and medical expenses, whether present or future. The third type is *punitive* and goes beyond compensating the victim; it is imposed to punish the individual who is found responsible for harming a victim. Its idea is to deter others and to keep the perpetrator away from society to avoid further crimes. In health care, we may hear the expression "suing so one never practices again"—that would be punitive because it aims at an action that exceeds specific compensation.

TORT LAW

Two basic items of civil law that are of concern in the practice of dental hygiene are **torts** and **contracts.** Torts are civil wrongs. They can be either *intentional* or *unintentional*. In addition, they can be acts of *omission* (i.e., not doing something that should have been done). They can also be acts of *commission* (i.e., doing something incorrectly. **Negligence** is an example of an unintentional tort; a dental hygienist did not intend to harm the patient, but his or her action or inaction inflicted harm. Examples of intentional torts in which there is an intention to harm are assault and battery, misrepresentation, defamation, and breach of confidentiality.

Professional Negligence and Malpractice

Negligence is not performing a clinical action (prophylactic or therapeutic) at the reasonable and acceptable standards of the profession, with the result of harm to the patient. A mistake *without* harm does not constitute negligence. In dental hygiene practice, negligence may be an act of omission or commission. Both are considered negligence. **Professional negligence** is neglecting to perform a procedure or action that is part of standard of care—that is, doing or failing to do what a reasonable and prudent dental hygienist would do under the same circumstances. It may occur at any time during the various stages of patient care, including during assessment, treatment, and follow-up. **Standard negligence,** or ordinary negligence, does not involve patient care. According to Scott (2000), if a patient falls on a slippery floor in a hospital and is harmed, ordinary negligence is involved, since falling on a slippery floor can happen anywhere—inside or outside of a hospital—and does not involve direct patient care. Professional negligence, in contrast, involves patient care.

Professional negligence may be substantiated by an *expert witness.* An expert witness is someone who is highly knowledgeable in a specialized area. For example, if a dental hygienist was accused of not following universal precautions, an expert witness could be a representative from OSHA or a dental professional who publishes or teaches in the area of blood-borne pathogens. This expert witness could defend the actions of the *defendant* (the dental hygienist accused of causing harm) by stating that the appropriate measures and standard of care were used, or the expert witness could testify against the dental hygienist and speak on behalf of the *plaintiff* (the patient who was harmed and is suing for professional negligence) and state that appropriate measures and standard of care was *not* used. In the case of the slippery floor, one does not need an *expert* to determine that the floor was slippery. Ordinary eyewitnesses can attest whether it was slippery or not.

In some cases of professional negligence, an expert witness may not be needed. The evidence is presented under the doctrine of *res ipsa loquitur* (the thing speaks for itself). This would occur, for example, if an instrument tip broke and was left in the sulcus or if treatment was performed on the wrong tooth. In other lawsuits, evidence can be judged from what is presented, or *prima facie* (at first sight). At times, a patient may contribute to the negligence or harm; this is referred to as *contributory* negligence. The patient has not taken reasonable care to protect his or her safety and thus has *contributed* to the injury or harm. For example, the patient who did not take prophylactic premedication is contributing to the negligence of the dental hygienist who treats a patient without asking if the premedication was taken and harm is a result of not being premedicated. This can be an important legal defense for a dental hygienist whose patient was noncompliant with recommendations (Davison, 2000, p. 51).

Malpractice (bad practice) is professional negligence that causes *harm.* For malpractice to occur, it must be established that an individual, a patient, was actually *harmed due to lack of standard of care.* For example, treating a patient who needs prophylactic coverage with antibiotics without the proper premedication is in itself not malpractice as long as no harm occurred. However, failure to premedicate a patient who needs antibiotic coverage, which results in that patient developing bacterial endocarditis, is malpractice. Harm has resulted from not premedicating a patient at risk, which is failure to meet the standard of care for a patient who needs antibiotics before dental hygiene treatment.

There are three conditions necessary to prove malpractice. It should be understood that dental hygienists have a duty to deliver standard of care. The conditions are:

1. There was an act of omission or commission.
2. There was failure to satisfy standard of care.
3. There was harm or injury to the patient.

Causes of malpractice include ignorance, lack of skill, neglect in applying skills, professional misconduct, lack of fidelity in performance of professional duties, and practice contrary to established rules. Therefore, dental hygienists must insure that they give a high quality of care. Among the means of achieving this aim are continuing education courses, cardiopulmonary resuscitation (CPR) certification, using critical-thinking skills in judgments regarding patient care, and being always aware of the standards of care in our locale. Most importantly, dental hygienists should know when to refer a patient to the appropriate expert, because we cannot all be experts. In addition, dental hygienists may need to make decisions regarding patient care if their standard of care differs from the standard others involved in the treatment of patients, such as dentists.

Malpractice cases could often be avoided through better communication between the provider and the patient. Good communication can often prevent court cases when the outcome of treatment was not what the patient expected. Following the protocols of informed consent and the patient as a partner model, as discussed in Chapter 3, "Informed Consent," may prevent a patient from suing. Informed consent is both ethical and legal. Paige (1977) cites two reasons for suing: unreasonable patient expectations and impersonal care (i.e., provider showing no interest). Accusations of malpractice can be avoided by resolving disputes internally and early, maintaining a dialogue with patients, practicing quality record keeping, being open to offering a refund, and referring early in treatment to a more experienced specialist (Curley, 1997, p. 24).

Although the majority of dental hygienists work under the supervision of dentists, they may be charged with negligence. An example of negligence on the part of the dental hygienist would be failing to inform the patient and/or the dentist about periodontal condition (Paige, 1977, p. 167). Negligence could also be charged if the dental hygienist did not provide standard of care, such as by not following the universal precaution protocol, with the result of causing disease transmission. Failure to probe that leads to undetected periodontal disease is another example of negligence. Under the principle *respondeat superior*, the dentist, as employer and supervisor, may also be responsible for the actions of the dental hygienist. But this does not relieve the dental hygienist from the guilt of neglect. Even though the dentist may be accountable for the actions of a dental hygienist, the latter may still be named as codefendant. Thus it is very important that dental hygienists have their own malpractice insurance; this will be further discussed in Chapter 11, "Planning for the Future and Career Longevity."

Assault and Battery

Assault and **battery** are other examples of *torts*, or civil wrongs, and may be considered in either criminal or civil court. *Assault* is threatening to harm an individual. *Battery* is touching an individual with the intention to harm. **Technical assault** or **technical battery** may occur even in the absence of the intention to harm, if there is no permission to touch. For example, attempting to perform or actually performing treatment that the patient did not consent to is technical assault or technical battery. The terms technical assault and technical battery may be used interchangeably. For example, applying a desensitizing agent to a tooth or a topical anesthetic to gingival tissue may be considered technical battery if the patient was not informed that this may be part of dental hygiene debridement therapy, although the intent is to make the patient more comfortable. A good rule is to always tell the patients what you are doing and why, so they can agree to each procedure. What may seem a routine act to the clinician may not seem routine to patients. This is why patients expect and deserve informative explanations.

Accusations of technical assault or technical battery can be avoided by obtaining informed consent. In our example, the patient did not give implied or expressed consent to topical anesthesia. The patient can argue that he or she gave no authorization to perform a procedure that was not mentioned. In that case, giving topical anesthesia without prior consent amounts to assault. The situation would be even worse for the dental hygienist if the topical anesthetic caused an adverse reaction, the possibility of which the patient was not informed of in advance. However, some states my consider lack of informed consent disclosure as negligence or malpractice, and not as assault and battery (Litch & Liggett, 1992; Rossoff, 1981).

Defamation

A third possible tort that may occur in dental hygiene practice is **defamation.** *Defamation* is making false statements that harm an individual's reputation. Defamation involves communication to a third person. Criticizing the treatment provided by another dental hygienist directly to that dental hygienist is not defamation. However, falsely criticizing the treatment provided by another dental hygienist to someone else (i.e., another dental hygienist, a dentist, a patient) is defamation. There are two types of defamation. **Libel** is written or published defamation. **Slander** is verbal defamation. Although it is unethical to criticize another professional's care to a patient, it may also be a *civil* wrong if the criticism is untrue.

Frequently, dental hygienists may be in a position to criticize the standard of care given to patients provided by another dental hygienist or dentist. However, we need to be cautious, as we do not know the circumstance in which the care was given and to what degree the patient may have contributed to the alleged negligence. Perhaps the patient never returned for follow-up appointments, or the dental hygienist faced problems beyond his or her control. In addition to written and verbal false statements, defamation may also occur with the inappropriate release of inaccurate medical information (i.e., patients' charts).

CONTRACT LAW

Contracts are agreements and obligations. The two types of *contracts* are implied and expressed. *Implied* contracts are assumed contracts; the parties need not have discussed the agreement in detail but showed interest in making a contract. For example, a patient sitting in the dental hygienist's chair and the dental hygienist providing treatment shows an interest in a contract between the dental hygienist and the patient; the patient will receive treatment and the dental hygienist will give treatment. *Expressed* contracts are verbally stated or written agreements by the involved parties. Courts have found that even a phone conversation between a provider and a patient constitutes a contract. Treatment plans are good examples of expressed contracts. Contracts are binding under three conditions: (1) the parties must be competent, (2) specific acts must be mutually agreed upon, and (3) there is a promise of something (i.e., payment for dental hygiene procedures) in return for something else (i.e., dental hygiene services). Situations that legally require written consent include trying new drugs, experimenting new procedures, taking a patient's photograph, giving general anesthesia, treating minor children in public programs, and providing treatment for more than one year. It may be helpful to review Chapter 3, "Informed Consent."

A patient arriving for a dental hygiene appointment is giving consent or agreement to have dental hygiene therapy. The agreement is usually that the dental hygienist will provide specific treatment and the patient will pay for these dental hygiene services. In dental hygiene, a *breach of contract* occurs when (1) financial rights or privacy rights have been violated, (2) services agreed to are not performed, or (3) services are delayed for an extended period of time. Harm *does not* have to occur for there to be a breach of contract. Under contract law, the dental hygienist, as a health care provider, has duties to the patient. These duties are outlined in Table 5–2. As you can see, many of the duties to a patient considered in a legal contract are also within the domain of acting ethically and following the ADHA Code of Ethics. Many of these duties, such as keeping accurate

Table 5–2   Duties of a Dental Hygienist as a Health Care Provider

To be licensed

To provide standard of care

To obtain informed consent

To keep current with treatment modalities

To render treatment within a reasonable time

To refer when necessary

To charge a reasonable fee

To treat within the scope of practice

To keep accurate records

To achieve a reasonable therapeutic or clinical result

To provide patient instructions

To inform patient of unexpected occurrences

To maintain confidentially

To not abandon the patient

To observe the fiduciary relationship created with the patient to maintain trust

To exercise reasonable skill, care, and judgment in diagnosis and treatment

---

records and other legal documents, will be covered further in this chapter and in Chapter 9, "Technology and Dental Hygiene."

Abandonment

One of the duties of the provider is nonabandonment, except in specific situations allowed by law. A health care provider cannot **abandon** a patient, that is, terminate treatment or refrain from seeing the patient, unless certain criteria are met. The provider-patient relationship can be *legally* terminated if (1) care is no longer needed, (2) the patient withdraws from the relationship, (3) the care of the patient is transferred to another health care provider, (4) ample notice of withdrawal is given, or (5) the provider is unable to provide care (Miller & Hutton, 2000, p. 422–423). In dental hygiene practice a patient may be refused an appointment for a variety of reasons such as repeated last minute cancellations, not arriving for scheduled appointments, or noncompliance with home-care. Non-payment for services can be a valid reason for ending a relationship (Darby & Walsh, 1995, p. 1083; Dietz, 2000, p. 57). However, Davison (2000) suggests that the health care professional complete all treatment started, even if the patient is not paying for services, and that he or she continue follow-up care of the patient until the threat of postoperative complications has passed (p. 80–81).

To legally terminate the dentist/dental hygienist–patient relationship, certain steps must be followed to prevent the liability of abandonment. The patient has to be told *in writing* that the dentist or dental hygienist is terminating the relationship, and the reasons should be provided. In addition, the letter should clarify that a copy of the patient's file will be sent to another dentist or dental hygienist upon written and signed request, and a list of other providers of dental or dental hygiene care should be given to the patient. Furthermore, the patient needs to be told what, if any, further treatment needs to be performed by the prospective providers. Such a letter should be sent by certified or registered mail with a return receipt requested; both the letter and returned receipt should be kept in the patient's file. The patient must be given a sufficient time (i.e., 30 days or more) to locate another dentist or dental hygienist to provide treatment. During this transitional period, emergency treatment must be rendered when needed.

Abandonment can also occur if the health care provider does not arrange for coverage during absence. It is essential that a dentist or dental hygienist provide information about how to seek help during his or her absence. For example, the dental office may have a phone message on the answering machine that directs a patient to call a certain number in case of emergency (i.e., gives dentist's home phone number or directs the patient to call another dentist or seek treatment at a specific facility). Also, the provider should inform the patient about where to seek care if there is a planned absence (i.e., vacation, hospitalization) shortly after procedures that may need emergency follow-up treatment, such as after periodontal surgery or tooth extraction.

Risk Management

Risk management is the term used to describe the actions taken to prevent financial loss or possible legal actions. Scott (2000) defines risk management as "the process of systematically monitoring health care delivery activities in order to prevent or minimize financial losses from claims or lawsuits arising from patient care or other activities conducted in a health care facility" (p. 191). Two basic areas of risk management in the dental office are record keeping and informed consent (Bressman, 1993, p. 63). Dental hygienists can avoid court cases by knowing the law and applying it. Ignorance of the law *does not* render one immune to it. In addition to good communication, the best protection from lawsuits is documentation. Records should be dated, signed, legible, and written in black or blue ink. Mistakes should never be whited out, but crossed out with a line, and an explanation given for the change. In a court case it is the defendant (i.e., the provider or dental hygienist) that needs to prove the absence of guilt. Individual states have laws regarding how long records need to be kept (i.e., 7 years, 10 years). Also, there are laws regarding the statute of limitations, that is, the length of time after an injury or damage in which a patient can sue or file a lawsuit. More information on risk management and quality assurance will be discussed later in the book.

LICENSURE

Educational Requirements

As stated earlier, licensure is a governmental regulation. Usually, licensing laws have educational and examination requirements. An individual must graduate from an accredited dental hygiene program. **Accreditation** status means that the program has met the minimal requirement standards outlined by the American Dental Association (ADA) Council of Dental Accreditation. These standards cover all phases of a dental hygiene program, from how students are admitted to patient confidentiality. Not only the academic component of the curriculum, but also other aspects that influence the curriculum, including faculty, facilities, and finances, are judged. The areas evaluated are (1) institutional effectiveness, (2) educational program, (3) administration, faculty, and staff, (4) educational support services, (5) health and safety provisions, and (6) patient care (Commission on Dental Accreditation, 1998). Through accreditation, dental hygienists and the public are guaranteed that minimal educational standards are met for the practicing dental hygienist. Although dental hygienists may participate in accreditation site visits to dental hygiene programs, the dentists still control the education of dental hygienists because programs are accredited by the ADA, and not by the ADHA.

Currently, Alabama is the only state that allows educational requirements to be attained through **preceptorship,** or on-the-job training. However, it is being discussed in other states. Dental hygiene preceptorship is the training of dental hygienists in the dental office by a dentist. Although there may be some official classroom requirements, such as basic sciences and clinical lectures, preceptor programs are not housed in an institution of higher learning. A dentist in Alabama is able to train an individual in a private dental office to be a dental hygienist with no standardized pre-clinical or clinical instruction; however, there is a required number of patients to be treated and criteria for the mastery of skills (Curran & Darby, 1990, p. 293).

Written Board Exams

One must have graduated (or will graduate within a certain period of time) from an accredited dental hygiene program to be eligible to take the National Board Dental Hygiene Examination. The Joint Commission on National Dental Examination is the agency responsible for the development and administration of the National Board Dental Hygiene Examination. This Commission includes representatives from dental schools, dental practice, state dental examining boards, dental hygiene, and the public. In addition, a standing committee of the Joint Commission includes dental hygienists who act as consultants. For example, faculty of dental hygiene programs act as experts in specific content areas for the formulation of questions for test construction. This exam is a written evaluation of theoretical knowledge through recall and case-based multiple-choice questions.

Practical Board Exams

In addition to a written exam, dental hygienists may also be required to take a practical board exam. In this exam, dental hygienists are required to demonstrate competency in providing dental hygiene services such as recording medical histories, performing an oral examination, charting existing oral conditions, taking radiographs, probing, detecting and removing calculus, and polishing. There are differences among states in the content of board exams, and each state may vary in terms of the passing score necessary. For example, the North East Regional Board Exam (NERB) consists not only of a patient treatment portion, but also a computer-simulated exam portion. This portion of NERB is called the computer-simulated clinical exercise. It is taken via a computer that displays slides illustrating various clinical topics and clinical situations. For example, the candidate may be asked to name an anatomy structure found on a radiograph. A state may have its own board exam, as do North Carolina and Indiana. Alternatively, a state may elect to participate with a group of neighboring states and recognize a regional board exam. In the case of regional board exams, states contract with nonregulatory testing agencies or for-profit testing services to administer clinical examinations. The regional board exams are North East Regional, Central Regional,

Southern Regional, and Western Regional. Information regarding these board exams is found in Appendices B and C.

Other Requirements for Licensure

As a student, you will decide where you plan to practice and take the practical board exam necessary for that state. Requirements for licensure are in a constant state of flux, and what was a requirement when you started dental hygiene may not be required now. Unfortunately, there are reciprocity restrictions. In other words, although the national written board is recognized throughout the United States, practical boards are not. If a practicing dental hygienist moves from one state to another, there is no automatic transfer of license. For instance, a dental hygienist who wants to practice in California needs to take the California Board even though he or she is licensed in Illinois through the North East Regional Board or the Central Regional Board. In addition, the dental hygienist who moves to California is required to take an examination (with proof of required education) for local anesthesia, which is a legal function for dental hygienists in California, but not in every state.

Although an individual state may recognize a regional board, it may have additional requirements for licensure, such as an examination covering the state dental practice act, continuing education courses in a specific area (i.e., child abuse, OSHA, nitrous oxide), or CPR certification. Dental hygiene, along with dentistry, is one of the few professions that require practical examination as well as written examination. For example, nurses pass a national theory exam but do not need to take a practical exam. In others words, they are not tested on nursing procedures such as taking blood pressure or changing a dressing. Some feel that this restriction on portability (relocation from state to state) is to protect the public; others feel that it is financially protecting those in the field by preventing an oversupply to an area; and others feel that it is a way one profession, dentistry, can have control over another profession, dental hygiene.

Credentialing

Another way to receive a license is through **credentials,** or credentialing. Credentialing is determined by each state. Usually, dental hygienists practicing specific procedures prior to the introduction of exams for those procedures are recognized as competent and are "grandfathered" into the profession and granted licensure. Another way to credential is to document that the dental hygienist is equal in skills to those presently licensed.

For example, a dental hygienist licensed in Ohio for many years may be granted a license in Illinois without additional examination requirements. The grounds for granting credentials may include a dental hygiene employment history signed by former employers or supervising dentists, a dental hygiene diploma, national board exam results, an active license elsewhere, good standing with other dental hygiene licensing agencies, and continuing education credits. Individual state dental practice acts usually have a section regarding reciprocity and credentialing.

Certification

A term often confused with licensing is certification. As already stated, the government grants license. Not all dental hygienists who are licensed are certified. Certification is granted by a nongovernmental entity such as an organization, institution, agency, or association. For example, dental hygienists may take an expanded function course (i.e., restorative, orthodontic, local anesthesia, nitrous oxide sedation). The certification is recognition that the dental hygienist had advanced training to perform these duties, but not the license to perform these duties.

STATE DENTAL PRACTICE ACT

The state dental practice act is statutory law, passed by legislatures, that controls the practice of dentistry and dental hygiene. It outlines the rules and regulations as interpretations of the law. In the state dental practice act, procedures are stated in regards to what a dental hygienist can and cannot do. These may be a "laundry list" of itemized procedures, or the act may use general statements that define the procedures that dental hygienists may perform (i.e., preventive services) and those procedures reserved for only dentists (i.e., diagnosis). The act also sets forth the educational requirements for dental hygienists, including continuing education. The purpose of the state dental practice act is to protect the public, and depending upon how the act is written and interpreted, it may also protect dentists and dental hygienists. Because the act is a law, it means that only those who abide by the act will be able to *legally* practice dental hygiene. Thus, unqualified personnel are prevented from jeopardizing the health of the consumer. Copies of the act were hard to obtain, and some states charged a fee for copies. However, each state's dental practice act is now accessible on the Internet. You will find links to each states's act at *www.adha.org* and *www.ada.org*.

Regulation

The dental profession regulates the majority of dental hygienists in the United States through dental boards. Members of these boards are appointed by the governor and may consist of dentists, dental hygienists, consumers, and other members of the dental team. In the past, dental hygienists did not have voting rights on some dental boards. Dental hygienists are now viewed as equal members on these boards, although in many instances they are still outnumbered by dentists. New Mexico and Washington are two states that have self-regulation; that is, they have authority in the regulation of dental hygiene. Other states have dental hygiene committees that make recommendations to the dental board. In addition, some states work with another nondental agency to regulate dentistry and dental hygiene. For example, in Illinois, the Department of Professional Regulations actually grants the license to practice dentistry and dental hygiene. Regulatory information on individual states can be obtained from the ADHA, ADA, and individual state dental and dental hygiene associations.

Changes in state dental practice acts are also made by legislation and are introduced as a bill. Then, according to legislative measures, the bill must be passed in both the House and the Senate. Either the House or the Senate can stop a bill or amend it. A bill can also be sent to a specially formed committee to modify the areas of disagreement between the House and Senate. The modified version is again reviewed by the House and the Senate. If the bill passes, it is given to the governor to either sign or veto. The bill can also become law without the governor's signature; however, it is better to have the governor's signature. It is very important during the time a bill is being considered that dental hygienists lobby. If a proposed bill would transfer dental hygiene functions to a less qualified group of practitioners, for example, and we, as dental hygienists, disagree with that bill, we should contact the legislators to express our concerns. We should resist any attempt by any other group working in the dental field to take over functions from dental hygienists, since that may jeopardize the dental hygiene profession. Legislators can be contacted by individuals or through a dental hygiene association. It is useful for the dental hygiene profession to employ lobbyists who can effectively contact legislators and persuade them to vote a certain way—the way that ensures protecting the public as well as the interests of the dental hygiene profession. Dental hygienists can also participate in lobbying through activities such as writing editorials and informative articles in newspapers, meeting face-to-face with legislators, and working on campaigns to establish links with legislators. Being politically alert and active is essential for protecting the rights of our profession.

Scope of Practice

Most state dental practice acts have a list of functions that dental hygienists can perform. Some dental hygienists feel that an official list is restrictive to dental hygiene and implies that dental hygienists cannot do those procedures not specified in the list. Others feel that the list protects dental hygienists because it entails that no other dental team member is allowed to perform the functions allocated for dental hygienists. Some states have *open provisions* that allow the dentist to determine which functions dental hygienists can perform. In these circumstances, the dental hygienists are usually not allowed to perform those functions reserved for dentists, such as diagnosis, cutting tissue, and writing prescriptions (Davison, 2000, p. 105).

Supervision

Dental hygiene is one of the few professions that require supervision from another profession. In fact, supervision is one of the features that prevent dental hygiene from being recognized as a full (or true) profession by some individuals and various organizations. A few states (e.g., California and Colorado) allow independent practice or unsupervised practice; however, specific functions need supervision by a dentist. For example, in Colorado a dentist's physical presence is required for the administration of local anesthesia and nitrous oxide. In many cases, lesser supervision is needed in public health settings or institutions. For example, dental hygienists in Illinois can treat nursing home residents without the physical presence of a dentist. However, the dentist must have examined the patient and provided written orders within 90 days before the initiation of dental hygiene treatment, and the dental hygienist must review the medical history and perform an exam (Illinois Department of Professional Regulations, 2000).

Some states allow pit and fissure sealants to be done without supervision; other states require a dentist to be present. A state may require the dentist to be physically present if the sealant is applied in private practice but not in other health care settings or on Native Indian reserves. Table 5–3 defines the four basic levels of supervision applicable to dental hygiene practice. Some states have additional restrictions on practicing without a

Table 5–3 Levels of Supervision in Dental Hygiene Practice Settings

General Supervision Practice	The dentist authorizes the procedures. The dentist does not have to be physically present.
Indirect Supervision Practice	The dentist authorizes the procedures. The dentist is physically present.
Direct Supervision Practice	The dentist authorizes the procedures. The dentist is physically present. The dentist approves the work after completion.
Unsupervised Practice	No supervision by dentist. No authorization by dentists.

dentist. For example, in Ohio a dental hygienist may qualify for approval to work without the dentists being physically present in the private dental office setting. This approval is based on years of experience, a course in identification and prevention of medical emergencies, certification in CPR, and a statement from a licensed dentist that the dental hygienist is competent to work without supervision. But there are restrictions to this mode of practice. For instance, it is allowed for no more than 15 consecutive working days (or three consecutive weeks of five working days per week). There are also set time limits for examination of patients by dentists before dental hygiene treatment, and the dental hygienist should comply with the dentist's written orders. In addition, it must be documented that the patient was informed that the dentist would not be present during dental hygiene treatment (Ohio State Dental Board, 2000). In these circumstances, the patient would be able to choose between supervised and unsupervised dental hygiene treatment.

SUMMARY

The practice of dental hygiene involves not only the ethical considerations discussed in the previous chapters but also legal considerations. Dental hygienists not practicing in accordance with the state dental practice act, which is legislated law, may be liable in criminal court. Dental hygienists may also be liable in civil court if they commit actions against individuals such as malpractice, defamation, technical assault, and breach of contract. With the exception of Alabama, dental hygienists must graduate from an accredited dental hygiene program and pass both a written exam and practical exam to be licensed. State dental practice acts outline the rules and regulations for the practice of dental hygiene. Levels of supervision vary according to the state, the procedure, and the treatment setting.

SELF-TEST

1. An illegal act against society is subject to criminal law procedures.
   a) True
   b) False
2. Torts are considered _____ wrongs.
   a) criminal
   b) civil
   c) medical
   d) none of the above
3. Damages in civil court cases may be _____.
   a) punitive
   b) compensatory
   c) nominal
   d) all the above
4. Written defamation is considered libel.
   a) True
   b) False
5. A _____ is a civil wrong or action that brings harm to an individual's person, property, or reputation.
6. Malpractice may be considered a tort because it causes ____ to an individual.
7. Negligence is a form of _____.

ACTIVITIES

1. Compare two state dental practice acts. What similarities do you find between the two acts regarding the practice of dental hygiene (i.e., continuing education requirements, supervision level, allowable procedures, fee payment, licensing body, etc.)? Report the findings to the class.

2. Debate the issue of levels of supervision found in a practice act. Do you feel one standard is appropriate for one setting and not for another? Why do you think a dental practice act is written with the various levels of supervision?

CASE STUDY

Scenario: You have just graduated from a dental hygiene program, moved to another state, and are currently employed by a periodontist. You have an 8-year-old son who has just started in a new school that requires a dental exam for enrollment. You make an appointment with a general dentist, recommended by your new employer, for your son's dental exam. You think this might also be a good time to establish a relationship with a general dentist for your family in this new area. In the past, you have done all the preventive work necessary for your son as a patient in the dental hygiene student clinic. Right before you graduated a few months ago, you did the following procedures: reviewed medical history, recorded intraoral and extraoral findings including the retention of sealants, exposed bitewing radiographs, reviewed toothbrushing, performed minimal debridement, selectively polished, and applied fluoride. You have brought a duplicate set of the recently taken x-rays, along with the school's enrollment form and your insurance form, and have given them to the receptionist.

You, your son, and the staff agree that your son should go to the treatment area alone. You have no problem with this decision, as you are aware that children may behave better without their parents and you are teaching your son to be independent. You wait in the reception area. Your son returns carrying the infamous toothbrush and wearing a sticker. As you sign the insurance papers and write the copayment check, you realize your son has had a dental exam along with polishing (prophy), two bitewing radiographs, and a fluoride treatment. A member of the staff has recommended sealants be redone. You ask to speak with the dentist because you would like to introduce yourself, and because this visit was to be only an exam. You would like an explanation why the other procedures were performed. You are told that the dentist has left the office but that he did see your son for the exam; the dentist will be back in the office after lunch. The school's enrollment form has been stamped with the dentist's name, phone number, and address. The receptionist initials it. You are aware of the state dental practice act, having just reviewed it for your own license as a dental hygienist. You know that dental hygienists in this state work with indirect supervision and dental assistants work with direct supervision. You ask to speak with the person who treated your son. You are told that your son was originally scheduled with the dental hygienists, but she was running late, so the dental assistant treated your son. You also know that polishing and fluoride are not within the scope of practice for dental assistants in this state.

How are you going to handle this situation, which seems to be illegal in many ways?

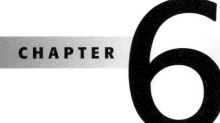

Social Issues

Upon reading the material in this chapter, you will be able to

1. Identify legislation that protects and aids the patient and the dental hygienist against discrimination in dentistry.
2. Recognize the signs of abuse (child, spouse, and elderly).
3. List barriers to access to care.
4. Discuss the advantages and disadvantages of various reimbursement or insurance plans (Medicaid, Medicare, and managed care) as they pertain to access to care and distributive justice issues.

As we have seen, ethical and legal issues often overlap. An issue can be both ethical and legal. Similarly, ethical and legal issues can also be integrated into social issues. Social issues that dental hygienists must sometimes deal with are related to obligations to society and to the problems of the workplace. Among the social issues addressed in this chapter are employment laws, reporting of abuse, and access to care. In addition to laws that govern the practice of dental hygiene and patient treatment that were discussed in Chapter 5, "Jurisprudence," there are federal and state laws that protect individuals in the workplace. Violations of these laws or acts can be judged throughout the various levels of the judicial system. Antidiscrimination laws not only protect the dental hygienists in the workplace, but also enable patients to receive equal quality of care. Another social issue that involves both ethical and legal responsibilities is the ability to recognize and the mandate to report abuse. Access to care is a social issue with legal and ethical ramifications. Barriers to access to care are financial, geographic, organizational, and sociological.

WORKPLACE LEGISLATION

There are both federal and state laws to protect employees. Unfortunately, some laws do not apply to dental hygienists due to the small number of employees working at a private dental office, the employment setting for the majority of dental hygienists. Frequently, where a federal law may not apply, a state may protect the sole employee. The appendix lists a few sources for more information regarding employment rights. A portion of this chapter will discuss some workplace laws that pertain to the dental hygiene practice. There are many other legal regulations that are applicable to dental hygienists, including minimum wage, unemployment and retirement benefits, taxes, and employment contracts. These will be discussed in Chapter 10, "Seeking the Dental Hygiene Position" and Chapter 11, "Planning for the Future and Career Longevity."

Affirmative Action

According to Title VII of the Civil Rights Act of 1964, an individual cannot be discriminated against because of race, color, religion, national origin, gender, or pregnancy. This act applies to the treatment of patients; that is, a health care provider cannot refuse treating a patient based on these criteria. This act also protects the dental hygienist as an employee. If a dental hygienist feels that he or she is discriminated against, the individual should contact the Equal Employment Opportunity Commission. Examples of discrimination include unfair denial of a job, denial of a deserved promotion, or not getting equal pay.

Dental hygienists may be especially vulnerable to discrimination in the private dental practice setting because they often rely on one person for employment: the dentist. In private offices that employ few workers, there are no strict regulations for hiring, promoting, or rewarding employees as there are for large organizations. The dentist ultimately decides who gets hired, the working conditions, and salary. Dental hygienists in private practice may find themselves in a difficult situation, where one person has the authority of making all decisions that affect their careers. For example, two dental hygienists working in the same office and doing equal work in terms of patient treatment may not be paid the same salary. Although there is a moral obligation for the dentist to do so, there is no legal process to ensure equal pay, particularly in practices that employ only a few dental hygienists. It may also happen that one dental hygienist has more experience or more education: In that case, should he or she be paid more? Again, what one dentist does, another may not, and there are no rigid rules to be followed.

Other situations may also raise questions about discrimination in the private office. What happens, for instance, if the male dental hygienist in the office does equal work but receives a higher salary? Also, as a dental hygienist gets older, would it be justified to replace him or her with a younger person? There are no strict guidelines to address such practices, but the dental hygienist who is treated unfairly may sue. The problem is that in employment settings involving a small number of workers, Affirmative Action is not always applicable. This, however, does not mean that dental hygienists are totally powerless. They can appeal to courts of law for correcting discriminatory practices.

Pregnancy Discrimination Act

Dental hygienists are especially vulnerable to pregnancy discrimination. A woman cannot be fired or denied a job because of pregnancy, childbirth, or related medical conditions, according to the Pregnancy Discrimination Act of 1978. If her pregnancy limits her job function, she must be granted the same job considerations as others with similar limitations or abilities. While on pregnancy leave, the employee must receive the same benefits given to other employees on leaves (i.e., vacation, pay increases, seniority). This act is very important for dental hygienists because it prohibits an employer from forcing a pregnant dental hygienist to take maternity leave either before or after birth. It also imposes an obligation on the employer to hold the job open for the same length of time as for other employees on sick or disability leave. A dentist could replace the dental hygienist while she is on maternity leave, and that is not against the law as long as it is a temporary replacement. But the law forbids permanent replacement of a pregnant employee.

Family and Medical Leave Act

This federal act, referred to as FMLA, allows leaves of absence of up to 12 unpaid weeks of salary for the employee after using all vacation pay and sick leave. Leave of absence is applicable for birth or adoption, serious illness, or care of a family member. Dental hygienists, the majority of whom are women, often have family responsibilities, commitments, and obligations that are protected by this act. Women are the ones who are usually expected to care for children as well as for sick family members. This law covers full-time workers in workplaces with 50 or more employees. Thus family medical leaves may not be applicable to the majority of dental hygienists. In fact, only those who work for organizations (e.g., companies, hospitals, government agencies, public health departments, educational institutions) can benefit from this law.

Americans with Disabilities Act

There are two sides to disability. First, disabled patients should not be discriminated against. Second, disabled dental hygienists should be protected from discrimination in the workplace. A disability is a condition that interferes with life function. In dental hygiene practice, care providers cannot withhold treatment or provide less quality of treatment to a disabled patient. This would be discrimination. However, we must recognize the difference between treating a patient with a disability and treating a medically compromised patient who may need to be treated in special facilities or by specialists. At times, there is a need to use different procedures for disabled patients in order to provide quality of care and standard of care. For example, a patient with AIDS can be treated safely in a dental practice due to universal precautions, while a patient with hemophilia may need to be treated in a hospital if the procedure is invasive. We have an ethical duty to treat those in need of care, but at the same time, we cannot risk harm to a patient with a special condition, other patients, or personal risk to the provider.

The question to ask is this: Is the treatment to a disabled patient the same as to the nondisabled patients? For example, if the dental hygienist does not double-glove for all patients, then he or she should not double-glove for a medically compromised patient or a patient with a communicable disease. Although gloving does provide a barrier against infections, some providers prefer to double glove to decrease operator exposure and inner glove perforation during high-risk oral surgeries (Schwimmer, Massoumi, & Barr, 1994). To double glove based on the individual patient and not the procedure would be discriminatory. However, if the dental hygienist feels that the patient's health status would be compromised or does not have the skills, equipment, or experience to treat a medically compromised patient, and has consulted with the patient's physician, then referral could be justified (Weinstein, 1993, p. 84). Not only do health care providers have to treat the disabled, they have to provide accessibility. Dental offices should be accessible through wheelchair ramps and elevators. The more recently constructed or renovated operatories accommodate wheelchairs.

Now it is appropriate to examine the other side of the issue of disability, that is, how the Americans with Disabilities Act applies to dental hygienists in the workplace. The rights of the handicapped were protected by the Rehabilitation Act of 1973. At first, the act applied only to employers or institutions that contracted with the federal government or had received federal funding. Only the handicapped employees of these employers were covered by the act. Later, infectious diseases became recognized as handicaps. In 1990 the Americans with Disabilities Act applied the same standards as the Rehabilitation Act and extended it also to private employers not receiving federal funding.

As a small business, dental offices do not have to comply with all the provisions of the Americans with Disabilities Act in terms of hiring. However, a dental hygienist cannot be disqualified from a position based on a disability, such as being confined to a wheelchair, as long as the dental hygienist can perform the same duties. According to the act, it is the responsibility of the employer or business (for example, the private practice dentist) to make structural changes to the office or purchase any special equipment required for the disabled person to perform the job (Ganssle, 1995, p. 24).

In interviews with paraplegic dental hygienists, Seckman (2000) found that the foot-operated rheostat of the dental handpiece presents a major problem for them. However, dental equipment manufacturers are receptive to the idea of altering equipment for the disabled. In addition, asepsis (i.e., regloving) does not seem to be a problem if dental hygienists use electric wheelchairs and cover the joystick with a bag. Needed equipment can be obtained through various agencies such as the State Department of Vocational Rehabilitation. If a dental hygienist or any other potential employee feels discriminated against, an attorney should be consulted.

Age Discrimination

The Age Discrimination in Employment Act prohibits employment discrimination based on age in businesses employing 20 or more workers, so this act protects dental hygienists over 40 years of age only in large facilities. The problem is that the dental office usually does not have 20 or more employees and therefore is not included under this act. However, the Age Discrimination Act of 1975, a national law, prohibits discrimination on the basis of age in programs or activities receiving federal financial assistance, such as health care and human service providers. This law may cover more dental hygienists as they become employed in the nontraditional dental hygiene practice settings receiving federal funding.

Sexual Harassment

Sexual harassment is unwelcome or unwanted behavior or activities of a sexual nature that occurs between two or more individuals of unequal power. Because males usually have higher positions of power in the workforce, sexual harassment is considered a form of sex discrimination. Therefore, sexual harassment is a violation of the Civil Rights Act. Sexual harassment, as an amendment to the Civil Rights Act and according to the guidelines of the Equal Employment Opportunity Commission, applies only to employment settings of 15 or more employees. Consequently, dental hygienists working in small private offices are less protected.

In a study of Washington dental hygienists, over 25 percent of the respondents had experienced harassment by either dentists or patients, and 35 percent knew of other oral health care staff who had been harassed. In addition, 23 percent of those harassed terminated employment by resigning or quitting rather than by being fired (Garvin & Siedge, 1992, p. 183). Thus sexual harassment in the dental office may be between a male dentist who has power as employer and a female dental hygienist who is a subordinate employee; the harassment may also come from a patient or colleague of the opposite sex. It can be between a female dentist and a male dental hygienist or between two individuals of the same sex. There can also be informal sexual harassment, where there is no formal hierarchy of power, such as between two students or two coworkers of equal status. It is important to note that sexual harassment tends to be a repeated behavior. For example, a one-time comment made in a joke may not be considered harassment, but repeated unwelcomed comments of a sexual nature constitute harassment.

Documenting sexual harassment is very important and should include the nature and description of the offensive behaviors and the dates, times, and names. Also, it is important to inform the offending individual (the person doing the harassing) that the behavior is unwelcome and to tell the immediate supervisor of the incidents. In the dental office, the dentist is the supervisor, so if the dentist is the one doing the harassing, the dental hygienist should inform a partner or an associate in the dental office or the office manager (McKee, 2000). If another employee is harassing an individual while functioning under the terms of employment and the supervisor does nothing about it, the supervisor may be also held accountable or liable for the harassment through *respondeat superior* (see definition in Chapter 5, "Jurisprudence").

Occupational Safety and Health Act

This act ensures a safe and healthy environment for both the patient and the dental hygienist; however, it was originally designed to ensure a safe work environment and protection from hazards in the industrial workplace. Even before you started dental hygiene, and probably as a requirement for dental hygiene, you followed procedures outlined in the Occupational Safety and Health Act (OSHA). For example, your dental hygiene program may have asked for proof of Hepatitis B vaccine and a tuberculosis test. Later in your dental hygiene studies, you received training in universal precautions, blood-borne pathogens, and OSHA guidelines. In your dental hygiene clinic, you may have used ergonomic operator chairs or stools. All these measures are enforced in order to follow protocols set by OSHA. These guidelines may remain the same or may change as you continue in dental hygiene or switch careers.

By law, dental hygienists are required to receive initial and annual updated training in OSHA, provided at the expense of employers and during working hours. Because private dental offices have less than 15 employees, these workplaces are not routinely inspected. But if OSHA guidelines are not followed in a dental office, regardless of the number of employees, a complaint can be filed and the dental office will be investigated.

An important aspect of occupational safety for dental hygienists is the role of ergonomics. Dental hygienists are prone to develop carpal tunnel syndrome as a result of the repetitive nature of dental hygiene procedures. This syndrome affects people who perform repetitive movements with their hands. Other musculoskeletal disorders may be preventable or lessened with good positioning and by following OSHA ergonomic standards that directly relate to the specific job activities of the dental hygienist.

Part of occupational health and safety in the workplace is protection against workplace violence. According to the National Institute for Occupational Safety and Health, homicide is the leading cause of workplace death among females. The most common reasons are robbery and disgruntled spouses. With more dental offices providing care at night, dental hygienists are at some risk for violence in the workplace as dental offices have money and drugs. It has been reported that health care facilities are a primary target of violence, especially by drug seekers. The best way dental hygienists can protect themselves and others against workplace violence is to use common sense. For example, if the office has a back door, it should be kept locked. Dental hygienists should also be aware of patients who are not happy with the services or treatment they have received, because they may translate their frustration into violence.

REPORTING DOMESTIC VIOLENCE

Domestic violence is family violence, violence that occurs in the home or within the family. Using this broad definition, the three types of domestic violence are child abuse, spouse abuse, and elderly abuse. Abuse can also occur outside the home—for example, in facilities such as day care and nursing homes. At times, the term *domestic violence* is reserved for spouse abuse. It is the dental hygienist's ethical and legal responsibility to recognize the signs of abuse and to report cases of abuse to the authorities in accordance with the regulations.

Child Abuse

Child abuse is any act that endangers or impairs a child's physical or emotional health or development. In most states dental hygienists, like other health care professionals, are mandated by law to report child abuse to governmental authorities. Many states, in fact, require continuing education on the subject of child abuse. Dental hygienists should know the law and protocol for reporting child abuse. Even in cases of suspected child abuse, providers are given immunity from liability and can be prosecuted for *not* reporting child abuse (Saxe & McCourt, 1991). In addition, dental hygienists are ethically responsible for protecting these children under the principle of *beneficence,* to benefit the patient. Coalitions such as Prevent Abuse and Neglect through Dental Awareness (PANDA) have been instituted to increase awareness and education among dental health care providers, including dental hygienists.

Warning signs of child abuse are repeated injuries (multiple bruises), unusual sites for accidental bumps and bruises, inappropriate behavior by the child, neglected appearance, strict, overly critical parents, and extremely isolated families. Sixty-five percent of all child abuse injures include trauma to the head, neck, or mouth (American Dental Association, 1998, p. 33). Therefore, dental hygienists and other dental health care providers are able to detect signs of child abuse. Indications of child abuse that are located outside the mouth include bruises, belt marks, cigarette burns, and bite marks. The most frequent oral injuries are fractured teeth, laceration of the lingual and labial frenula (frenum) due to forced feeding, missing teeth for which there is no obvious explanation, displaced teeth, discolored teeth, and abnormalities of appearance and mobility of the tongue. Other damage to the tongue, fractures of the maxillary and mandible, and bruised or scarred abrasions at the corners of the mouth are also common (da Fonseca & Idelberg, 1993, p. 136; Saxe & McCourt, 1991, p. 363). Signs of sexual abuse may also be found in the mouth: erythema and spetechiae of the palate as well as lesions of sexually transmitted diseases.

Signs of neglect, such as dressing a child for the wrong type of weather or lack of personal hygiene, may also be apparent. Child abuse can also include dental neglect, which is the willful failure of a parent or guardian to seek and follow through with treatment necessary to ensure a level of oral health essential for adequate function and freedom from pain and infections. This type of child abuse can be reported in the same manner as physical abuse. Caution should be used to avoid confusing signs of neglect with the inability to afford the cost of care or other barriers to access to care that are beyond the parent's control.

Documentation of abuse is important. In addition to recording in the child's chart a description of the injury (i.e., size, shape, location, color), a photograph should be taken. X-rays may also be taken, although that requires the permission of a parent or guardian. If taking a photograph is not possible, sketch the sign of abuse. In cases of suspected child abuse, parent permission may not be needed to take photographs and x-rays in some states. Dental hygienists should know what is legally allowed without parental permission according to the relevant state laws (e.g., health and safety codes, health practice acts, penal codes, child abuse reporting act). The practitioner should ask the child what happened (if possible, without the parent's presence) and then to ask the parent what happened. This should be done in a nonthreatening and nonaccusatory way, as the parent may not be aware of the abuse if it is from another caretaker. A threatening confrontation could also spark an angry reaction from the parent. However, hesitation or hostile answers from the parent, conflicting stories from the child and parent, or inconsistency between the parent's account and the injury may be cause for suspicion. For instance, an injury that is claimed to have happened yesterday would not be yellow in color; a yellowish color should raise the index of suspicion. The parent's and child's stories should also be documented. The dental health care provider may also consult with other health professionals, such as the family physician.

After reporting the incident to the proper authorities (e.g., state child protection agency or child abuse hotline) by phone, the dental health care provider may need to send the necessary documentation. It is important to be familiar with the reporting regulations in the state where you practice dental hygiene. Although it is the mandate of social services to investigate reported cases, the dental health care provider should follow up on the reported case of child abuse. The dental hygienist may discuss suspicions and precautions with the supervising or employing dentist before reporting child abuse. Some feel that reporting child abuse should be done when there is certainty, as it can be easily mistaken and its reporting can cause much distress and upheaval to the family. Others feel that any suspicion should be taken seriously. Dealing with individual cases requires using the prudent judgment of the dental hygienist. It is important to remember that even if the supervising dentist or other office personnel do not want to get involved, the dental hygienist has both a legal and moral duty to report child abuse.

Spouse Abuse

The term *domestic violence* covers spouse abuse, battering, or control over an intimate individual. **Spouse abuse** is an important form of domestic (same household) violence. It happens to women (as victims) more often than to men. As in the case of child abuse, there are laws in some states that require health care providers to report spouse abuse. However, reporting these incidents is more problematic than reporting incidents of child abuse because the suspected victim can sue for breach of confidentiality if he or she was not consulted first. The suspected victim may claim that the report was filed against his or her will. In this case there is not liability protection for the dental hygienist (American Dental Association, 1998, p. 23). Therefore, spouse abuse should not be reported without the consent of the abused spouse.

The majority of spouse abuse occurs with the female (battered woman). She may be abused by someone with whom she is has been intimate, such as a husband or a significant other. The abuse usually starts with controlling behavior from the abusive spouse; this behavior escalates and becomes more frequent and more aggressive. The dental hygienist should attempt to question the suspected abused patient away from the partner, document findings, speak to the patient in a nonjudgmental way, and have another staff corroborate any suspected findings. Following are examples of questions to ask the patient. Using the S.A.F.E. acronym, these questions are easily remembered. According to this acronym,

> S = Stress/Safety: *Does the patient feel safe? stressed? Is there a concern for safety?*
>
> A = Afraid/Abused: *Does the patient feel afraid? Has the patient or child been abused or threatened?*
>
> F = Friends/Family: *Do the family and friends of the patient know about the abuse? Will they give the patient support? How isolated is the patient?*
>
> E = Emergency Plan: *Does the patient have an emergency plan? Would the patient like to have one? Does the patient know where a shelter is located? Does the patient have a safe place and resources for an emergency?*

These are examples of questions that the dental hygienist may use in either a direct or indirect way (Ashur, 1993, p. 2367; Gibson-Howell, 1996, p. 79). The dental hygienist needs to be supportive when asking these questions and to act as a resource for the abused patient.

Among the signs of spouse abuse that can be identified by the dental hygienist are injuries involving the face, eyes, and neck. These may be detected during routine dental hygiene care. The health care provider should be suspicious of repeated bruises, broken bones, cigarette burns, human bite marks, and other signs similar to those found in child abuse. Again, it is very important to document cases of suspected spouse abuse. However, unlike child abuse, not all states have laws that mandate health care providers to report spouse abuse. But ethically, dental hygienists are required, through the principle of beneficence, to *benefit* the patient and promote the well being of the patient. So if reporting spouse abuse in a state is not mandated, the dental hygienist should offer advice and support.

Elderly Abuse

Another form of abuse is **elderly abuse.** This occurs when a relative (i.e., child, spouse, or other family member) or a health care provider abuses a geriatric patient. Elderly abuse can be physical, sexual, emotional, confinement, passive neglect, willful deprivation, and financial exploitation. The most common form of elderly abuse is financial. For example, a child, the primary care provider, or another person may cash the social security check of an elderly person and spend it for personal use rather than for the needs of the elderly individual.

More than half of the abusers are the primary caregivers (Elderly Abuse & Neglect Program, 1991). As with child and spouse abuse, dental hygienists should look for signs of physical abuse. These could include unexplained or unusual injuries, lack of appropriate dress or personal hygiene, and behavior that reflects abuse, such as being withdrawn or suspicious of the dental hygienist as a result of losing trust in others. Also, behavior of a caretaker who accompanies an elderly patient (i.e., not allowing older individual to speak for self) should raise suspicion (see Table 6–1). Suspected elderly abuse should be reported to the local social service agency that deals with aging or elderly abuse and neglect. In some states dental hygienists are mandated to report elderly abuse as they are to report child abuse. It is necessary to document findings similarly to child abuse and spouse abuse. As the elderly population grows and relies on primary care providers, it is important that the dental hygienist be aware of potential elderly abuse, its signs, and how to confront the situation legally and ethically.

One of the problems associated with reporting elderly abuse is that the elderly person may not want the dental hygienist to report the abuse. This can be a difficult situation. For example, if the abuser is a child of the abused, the elderly individual may not want to report the actions of the son or daughter. Also, elderly persons may think of the consequences of reporting abuse and worry about losing the sympathy of those who take care of them.

Many states have legislation that facilitates the reporting of elderly abuse. For example, the Illinois Elderly Abuse and Neglect Act protects reporters and caseworkers from civil or criminal liability (Illinois Depart-

Table 6–1   Some Common Signs of Abuse

Physical	Unexplained bruises
	Bruises at different stages
	Bite marks
	Injuries to head and face
Emotional	Withdrawn
	Lack of eye contact with abuser
Neglect	Dressed improperly
	Lack of personal hygiene
	Denied medical/dental care

ment on Aging, 1999). There are many local agencies available for support and information. In most situations, the local social service agencies can help the abused. If you cannot find a *local* agency that can help an elderly abused patient, contact the American Association of Retired Persons (AARP), a national advocate organization for senior citizens.

ACCESS TO CARE

Although the United States may be viewed as a country with good health care in terms of medical technology and skilled practitioners, Americans lack easy, affordable **access to care** (see Table 6–2). Access to care is an individual's ability to obtain timely personal health services to achieve the best possible health outcomes (Public Health Futures Illinois, 2000, p. 89). Other countries are able to provide more health services to more people and to have a healthier population at less cost. The problems with access to care apply also to oral health. It has only been in recent years that awareness of the dental needs of the American population have surfaced at a national level. Current studies have indicated that oral health is an indicator of overall health; research has shown correlation of periodontal disease with other health problems, such as heart disease and low-term birth rates (Loesche, 1997). Consequently, the status of dental health within a population is an indicator of status of general health in that population. The US Surgeon General's Report, released on May 25, 2000, included for the first time a report on oral health (US Department of Health and Human Services, 2000).

Justice

Earlier in this book, the concept of justice was discussed as an ethical consideration. Justice is a major factor in determining public policy. The allo-

Table 6–2 Access to Care Barriers

Financial	Money
	Insurance restrictions
Location	Travel restrictions
	Provider availability
Sociological	Perceived need
	Language

cation of health care resources, including oral health care, is among the prime objectives of public health policies. **Distributive justice** is concerned with how scarce resources are fairly distributed among members of the population. The allocation of resources can be based on the needs of an individual (microallocation) or the public (macroallocation). Distributive justice aims to allocate resources based on equality by rendering treatment facilities open to every citizen equally. It cannot be overemphasized that our society needs and desires eliminating the obstacles to affordable *access to care.* Justice should not be overlooked in such a project.

In addition to the importance of giving equal treatment to every person, treatment should also be based on need. That is, treatment should be given to all people who need it. Factors other than need include contribution and merit. People who are esteemed by society for their distinguished services, effort, or important contributions may be rewarded with preferential treatment (for a similar discussion see Darby, 1998, p. 765; and Munson, 1996, p. 38–40). For example, should all individuals be entitled to dental care, and should all dental care be equal? Does everyone have the *right* to the same dental care? Or, is dental care a *need,* and should those most in need have it first? Likewise, is dental care a *commodity,* and should only those who have merit (good qualifications) or the ability to afford the cost have it? The *egalitarian* would believe that equal treatment is a must for everyone. The *utilitarian* would try to allocate resources that would benefit the most while doing the least harm. The *libertarians* may propose that need is not a prime factor in the distribution of resources (Nelson, 2000, p. 580). Others believe that equals should be treated equally and unequals should be treated unequally. For example, one group of individuals should have access to costly implants while other groups can have bridges or partial dentures, each according to its ability to afford the cost.

A problem arises when the question of which group or individual should get the most expensive and effective alternative. Should those who are offered the implants be the ones who have financial resources or higher social positions, or those who are most valued in society? Should the element of compensation be taken into consideration? For example, should the person who had severe oral injuries as a result of cancer or an accident have a better form of treatment than an individual who lost tooth and bone structures due to periodontal disease from neglect? A similar question is whether the dental hygienist who has developed carpal tunnel syndrome from dental hygiene practice should be treated for it sooner and at a better level of care than another dental hygienist who developed carpal tunnel syndrome from leisure activities such as playing the piano?

Such questions fall in the realm of compensatory justice. Compensatory justice is concerned with compensations for wrongs that have been done (Purtilo, 1999, p. 60).

Another form of justice is procedure justice that concerns allocating resources in an orderly and impartial manner. Using the carpal tunnel syndrome example, if the leisure piano player was first in line for the operation, then the piano player would be operated on before the dental hygienist who acquired the disease from hard work. There are different views of distributive justice. Although the egalitarian view is the most ethical, it may be the most difficult to apply in practice because of the financial limitations. Yet we should aspire to adopt it as the basis for a better future system of oral health care.

Financial Barriers

One of the major barriers to access to care is the lack of financial resources. The uninsured cannot afford to be sick or to seek preventive services. It is alarming that the number of those without dental insurance is three times the number of those without health insurance. That is, access to dental care is much more limited than access to general health care. It is speculated that a universal health care system may solve the financial problem; however, it may not solve all the access problems, such as transportation, distance, lack of providers, and an individual's perceived need for treatment. Further measures need to be undertaken to facilitate access to oral health care. To enhance access to oral health care, strategies need to be developed that provide dental insurance as well as the means to obtain the care.

Traditionally, dental services, including dental hygiene services, were reimbursed through fee for service. The patient paid the dentist for the treatment received. Later, private dental insurance became available. In this financial arrangement, an individual would pay a premium to the insurance company, which would pay a portion of selected treatment costs, and the patient would pay the balance (called a copayment) and would also be responsible for the cost of procedures not covered by the insurance plan.

Although insurance may help relieve the financial barrier, the worry is that insurance dictates treatment. Based on the restrictions on reimbursement by insurance companies, a dentist may decide to use one type of restorative material or procedure that is less expensive than another, regardless of the long-term benefit to the patient. Also, patients may decide to visit dental hygienists once a year instead of twice or three times a year because the insurance will pay for only one visit each year. Similarly, if fluoride is not covered under the insurance plan, a parent may not give consent for a child to receive it. Insurance can also influence a wide range of policies in the dental office, from who gets a toothbrush to the length of an appointment. It may also affect referrals to a specialist, and some dental insurance plans restrict the care provided by specialists to the most complicated conditions. This is true not only for the dental but also the medical profession, where the physician or primary care provider is pressured to act as the *gatekeeper* for the insurance company and limits referrals to specialists. So, reducing financial barriers through insurance is not without its disadvantages.

Managed Care

Managed care, or health maintainance organizations (HMOs), are based on the strategy of lowering the cost of care by preventing disease and maintaining health. The idea behind managed care is to get individuals in good health and then to *maintain* that health so that the cost of treatment becomes more affordable. Managed care has evolved into a system of health care delivery that controls utilization and costs of services and measures performance to deliver quality, cost-effective health care (Public Health Future Illinois, 2000, p. 93). The three types of managed care plans for dentistry are dental health maintenance organization (DHMO), preferred provider organization (PPO), and capitation (Bergmann, 2000, p. 48). Managed care plans allow for greater access to care in terms of financial coverage for the patient, although managed care may limit the choice of providers.

Capitation is one form of managed care. In this financial system, the dentist contracts with the insurance company to provide services to a given number of individuals enrolled in the managed care program. The dentist receives a monthly payment based on the number of individuals. Two problems are associated with this plan. First, the patients are assigned to a certain dentist; thus a patient has a limited choice in selecting a dentist or is forced to receive care from only that dentist. Second, the dentist receives a set amount of money per patient; thus the dentist may be forced to use a lower standard of care in terms of cost for treatment procedures or to absorb the cost and lose money. For example, if a patient presents with a need for replacing several amalgam restorations, the dentist has to decide to use amalgam again or to use a higher cost esthetic material; obviously, financial factors will influence the decision. The advantage of capitation for the dentist is that it provides a guaranteed income over the whole year. Its advantage for patients is lower cost.

A DHMO is another form of managed care plan. In this plan a dentist provides all the services specified in the plan to individuals enrolled in the plan. In the third type of managed care, PPO, the patient selects a dentist from a given list of providers. The difference between these two plans and capitation is that the dentist is paid for procedures and not according to how many individuals are enrolled in the plan.

Although the American Dental Association is against managed care because it may control treatment of the patient and/or income of the dentist, the American Dental Hygienists' Association is in favor of managed care. Managed care could provide careers for dental hygienists, from traditional clinic dental hygiene practice in private dental offices to managed care centers. Also, more nontraditional roles could be created, such as quality assurance and management utilization review. In addition, dental hygienists are the preventive experts. If managed care organizations would pay a dental hygienist directly for the services rendered, rather than paying through a dentist, money could be saved for the insurance companies. The savings could be used to provide more preventive care to more individuals and to finance more restorative and other types of dental treatments.

Government Assistance

Medicaid covers indigent or low-income individuals; however, it does not cover preventive dental services for adults, which would include dental hygiene services. Each state determines how much it will reimburse the dentist for treatment, and this may be limited to emergency procedures or dentures. Under Medicaid, dental services are considered optional services. However, dental screenings are part of the Early and Periodic Screening Diagnosis and Treatment (EPSTD) covered by Medicaid for children. Dentists can elect to participate in Medicaid, but this is an optional choice. An individual may be covered by Medicaid for dental services without being able to obtain the needed dental treatment because the dentist does not accept Medicaid. It has been reported that only 20 percent of the Medicaid-eligible children actually receive preventive oral health services (Peck, 2000, p. 43). The reasons cited by the dental community for not accepting these patients are the low reimbursement by the government and the paper work involved (LeBlanc et al., 1997). Some dentists also state that cancellation of appointments, or *no shows,* by this segment of the population is another reason for not accepting Medicaid patients.

In an effort to reach children who may not have private insurance or the financial resources to pay for treatment, the government has instituted the Children's Health Insurance Program (CHIP) or State Children's Health Insurance Program (SCHIP). Each state has its own program under this plan. (See appendix for more information.) For example, in Illinois the program is *Kid Care*. The amount of the insurance premium is based on a sliding scale that considers the number of dependents and annual income of the family. This plan covers not only children but also pregnant women. This is an attempt by the government to provide health care for the uninsured working poor.

Medicare is the nation's largest health insurance program. It provides insurance coverage for individuals who are 65 years or older, who are disabled, or who have permanent kidney failure. Medicare provides both hospital and medical insurance; however, it does not cover prescriptions or any dental treatment, including preventive dental hygiene services. With an aging population and the high cost of prescription drugs, extended Medicare benefits has become both a social and political issue.

Location Barriers

Another barrier to access to care is location in terms of geography and organization. A geographic barrier is the distance from providers. This is especially true in rural areas where people may have to travel an hour or more to obtain care. In addition, location is a problem in rural areas because of the lack of a public transportation system (e.g., bus or metro lines). Some residents of rural areas do not have reliable cars or cannot afford the cost of gasoline. Therefore, an individual must have private means to reach a health care provider. Moreover, the elderly may be incapable of driving a private vehicle or using public transportation, and may have to rely on others for transportation.

In addition to geographic barriers, there are also organizational barriers—or lack of available providers. This is especially true in rural areas. The average traveling time in rural districts is estimated to be twice the length of the time in urban districts (Edelman & Menz, 1996). Twenty five percent of rural residents do not have a dentist available in close proximity, and in areas of health care provider shortage, 55 percent of the population do not have dentists within the same zip code area (Knapp & Hardwick, 2000, p. 45). One study (LeBlanc et al., 1997) reported that in some rural areas, people have to travel as far as three hours to obtain the necessary dental care. This same study reported that 63 percent of the respondents did not have a dentist in their town, and 45 percent reported that the nearest dentist was more than 20 miles away. In addition, there was a need to travel in excess of 90 miles to receive care from a dentist who accepted Medicaid. As discussed earlier, there is a problem with dentists accepting Medicaid patients, so there may be providers in a given area that do not accept Medicaid.

Furthermore, some areas have a low ratio of providers to population. An effort has been made by the federal government to provide oral care through the National Health Service Corps, where a health professional may work in an underserved area as part of a loan repayment for school. Unfortunately, there are not very many of these positions available for dental hygienists. And even if a dental hygiene student chooses to work in an underserved area after graduation, this may not be allowed when there is no supervising dentist in that area. An area may not be lacking in dental hygienists, but may have no dentists. In that case, the area would not be able to utilize dental hygienists because dentists are needed for supervision of the majority of dental hygienists. If the supervision laws were to change, dental hygienists would be able to serve more individuals and increase access to care. This would increase access not only in private practice settings but also in other areas, such as public health facilities, chronic care facilities, and even schools. For example, access to care for children could be increased if dental hygienists were allowed to perform preventive procedures such as pit and fissure dental sealants without direct supervision.

Sociological Barriers

Even if an individual is able to afford care through private or public means and there are providers available, this does not mean that this individual will seek the care or have easy access to care. People must not only have the means to obtain dental care, but should be motivated to receive care and to recognize the need for such care. So, another barrier to access to care is the perceived need for care. Those who do not believe in the importance of oral health and usefulness of a dental visit would not be willing to access dental care. This is especially true with preventive care. Many individuals do not seek care until they are in pain because they are unaware of the significance of preventive care. However, the availability of a regular provider increases the use of dental services because motivated persons would try to utilize any available services.

Another sociological barrier to access to care is discrimination. Previous discussion has shown how low-income Medicaid individuals are discriminated against by not being accepted by many dentists. Other discriminating factors can be associated with disabilities, and this is against the law. Many practitioners do not feel comfortable or competent with individuals who may be mentally or physically disabled; therefore, they may refer them to other providers who have more experience or willingness to deal with this group of patients. As a result, these disabled individuals may have limited access to care in the vicinity of their homes. In an effort to overcome this disparity and to encourage treatment of disabled individuals in their own vicinity, emphasis on training students to deal with disabled patients has been placed in the education curriculums of dental and dental hygiene programs. In addition, oral health care providers are encouraged to treat not only the disabled but also the elderly, the medically compromised, and other special populations in the private practice setting in order to increase access to care for these individuals. Likewise, some supervision laws for dental hygienists have been relaxed (i.e., from direct supervision to general supervision) so that individuals or residents in health care facilities can receive preventive dental hygiene care.

Language barrier is another factor that leads to limited access to care. This is especially true with the immigrant population. Newman & Gift (1992) found that ethnic minorities tend to utilize dental care facilities less than those from the ethnic majority. Moreover, immigrants may not know how to seek and obtain the necessary services that will increase their access to care. For example, they may not be aware of public health clinics if the advertisement is geared only to those who speak and read English. The population of the United States is becoming more diverse, and with this comes the need to communicate in a language other than English and to understand and respect cultural differences that relate to health care.

SUMMARY

Dental hygiene practice involves social issues that take into account both ethical and legal viewpoints. Three social issues that have legal and ethical ramifications are employment legislation, abuse reporting, and access to care. Dental hygienists are protected in the workplace by legislation; however, the employment laws may not always be applicable to the private dental office where the majority of dental hygienists work. Dental hygienists need not only to recognize abuse (child, spouse, and elderly) but also to help the abused individual through referring and/or reporting to the proper social service or legal authority. Access to care is hindered by financial barriers, location, lack of providers, and sociological factors.

Public policy such as government aid and supervision laws need to be changed to increase access to dental hygiene care.

SELF-TEST

1. The principle of distributive justice considers the allocation of health care resources according to an individual's (or group's)
   a) need.
   b) right.
   c) merit.
   d) all the above.
2. Universal health care would uphold the principle of distributive justice based on the theory that all individuals have an equal right to heath care.
   a) True
   b) False
3. Medicare, not to be confused with Medicaid, is designed for a specific segment of the population; this group is the _____.
4. Changing laws regarding the supervision of dental hygienists may increase access to preventive dental hygiene services to an underserved population because a _____ will not need to be present during treatment.
5. A major problem associated with Medicaid recipients receiving dental care is
   a) preventive care is not covered for adults.
   b) not all dentists accept Medicaid for payment of treatment.
   c) a and b.
   d) none of the above.
6. All access to care problems can be solved by decreasing the cost of care.
   a) True
   b) False

ACTIVITIES

1. Divide into all groups. Assign each group a different barrier to access to care. Brainstorm ideas that individual or groups of dental

hygienists can do to lessen or eliminate these barriers. Report back to the class.

2. Ask your friends and relatives to state the problems they have encountered in receiving dental or dental hygiene care. What solutions or suggestions are you able to offer to increase their access to dental and dental hygiene care?

3. Write a letter to the editor addressing the barriers to dental and dental hygiene care that you have observed in your community or with the patients you have treated in your program's dental hygiene clinic. Include recommendations.

4. Meet with your legislature to discuss how the state dental practice act needs to be changed to increase access to dental hygiene care for individuals living in your state or for a particular group of individuals who now have limited access to dental hygiene care.

CASE STUDY

Scenario: An individual does not have the financial means to seek regular preventive dental care. This individual is on Medicaid, which does not cover preventive dental hygiene care. Thus, caries are not detected at an early stage. The caries develop further, resulting in pain and loss of tooth structure. The patient now needs a root canal and a crown. However, the patient is still not able to afford dental care. There is no dentist in the area that will take Medicaid patients. This patient must travel two hours to get care from a dentist that will accept him as a patient. The dental office has told him that if he does not keep his appointment, another one will not be made for him. He does seasonal work and temporary work. He does not know when he will be called to work. If he keeps the appointment, he may lose a day's salary and not be able to work again for a while or may lose this job because he was not available that day. In addition, his friend will have to take a day from work to drive him to the dental office. The pain is so bad that the patient goes to the emergency room of a hospital three hours away, where the tooth is extracted.

What ethical and social problems are encountered by this individual? How can these problems be solved?

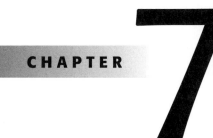

CHAPTER 7

Aspects of Practice Management

Upon reading the material in this chapter, you will be able to

1. Discuss the need for practice management in the dental office.
2. Identify different *management styles.*
3. Differentiate between oral health care and the business of oral health care.
4. Discuss the *team concept.*
5. Identify the benefits of *crosstraining.*
6. Differentiate types of *staff meetings.*
7. Differentiate between *employer expectations* and *employee expectations.*
8. Identify uses of *public relations* and *image* for the dental/dental hygiene practice.
9. Identify *patient needs* as they relate to dental hygiene.
10. Discuss how *marketing* relates to the dental/dental hygiene practice.
11. Identify advantages and disadvantages of *profit centers.*

Why is practice management included in the dental hygiene curriculum? Many new dental hygienists are unfamiliar with the everyday operations of the dental practice because they have no experience in a dental office as a dental assistant or office staff. Dental hygiene education has provided a strong foundation to delivering dental hygiene care. Yet there are numerous tasks to be completed by the office manager, the insurance processor, the dental assistant, and all other staff members employed in a practice. Each person has a specific set of duties unique to his or her position. Dental hygiene services are only a portion of what takes place in a dental office for patients to maintain optimal oral health.

Currently, several states, including Washington, Colorado, and New Mexico, have allowed dental hygienists to provide dental hygiene care under alternative practice settings, which include rehabilitation facilities, assisted and long-term care facilities, and free-standing dental hygiene practices. This means that with additional education and special licensure, the practitioner is able to practice in settings other than the dental office. Each state defines *alternative* or *independent* practice differently, and it is wise to consult with the licensing agency in any specific state. Understanding how a practice must operate in the business world will assist in its success.

Prior to the 1950s, dental students received no practice management information, and some of today's dental education programs neglect to include it. Dental students are taught theory and technical aspects of saving teeth and restorative dentistry, but without practice management information, new dentists may be overwhelmed by such tasks as ordering supplies, charging and billing patients, and hiring and firing employees.

During the 1970s and 1980s, dental schools began to understand the need to incorporate practice management courses into their curriculums. Still today, however, dental students and dental hygiene students are so focused on completing their requirements that it is difficult for school curriculum to include enough of this information (Miles, 1999). Time and the assistance of professional management consultants have contributed to an increase in management skills and business knowledge for dental graduates. Dentists and their practices are better prepared to succeed in the business environment.

In the early 1980s, the field of dentistry began to focus more on aesthetics and cosmetic procedures as a result of more people keeping their teeth longer. Again, many practices had difficulty showing a profit while providing these services. Remember that dental care resides in the health field, not the business field. Dentists would watch their **accounts receivables** rise out of control due to increasing fees and patients needing to finance their dental work. Dentistry is a health care profession whose main goal is to provide health care service. However, the dental practice is also a small business required to make a profit if it is to survive in the business world. At the same time, professional management consultants and firms began to capitalize on the need for business skills, knowledge, and operating systems in a dental practice that would increase profitability and decrease staff turnover.

The main objective presented by consultants was to have all staff members be accountable for their positions. Each member was seen as an important contributor to the team. By training staff to apply business theory, skills, and systems, the overall productiveness of the practice would benefit. Therefore, management consulting firms offered a business approach to operating the dental practice by involving the entire staff and incorporating systems designed to streamline the many tasks that take place on a daily basis. Some of the most notable management consulting firms include *Linda Miles, The Pride Institute,* and *McKenzie Management.* Many of these firms have been around for over twenty years, offering their expertise to dentists and their staff and incorporating systems designed to streamline daily tasks while the dental practice realizes a profit.

The practice of dental hygiene has seen similar concerns as dental hygienists enter into independent and alternative practice or obtain expanded licensure to include restorative procedures. Billing insurance, collecting fees, managing staff, and managing supplies are among the common obstacles that may affect the operational aspect of the practice. Lack of knowledge in financial management and accounting procedures also hinders immediate success for those who choose this career path. Although dental schools and dental hygiene programs continue to provide some practice management education for students, the actual implementation of this knowledge remains a challenge for many practitioners. Currently, there are numerous resources available to students and practitioners, for example, the American Academy of Dental Practice Administration and specialized publications that focus on practice management issues.

The use of a professional management consultant or firm may be advantageous to the dental practice and its team members to ensure longevity while providing quality dental care. However, not all management firms or consultants have the "cure all" solutions to any particular dental or dental hygiene office.

PROS AND CONS OF MANAGEMENT CONSULTANTS

When employers make the decision to hire a professional practice management consultant, the consultant requests participation by all staff members. The cost for a professional consultant generally runs high, and the training process may extend over a long period of time (months to years). The consultant presents ideas and systems that are designed to improve the practice in areas of patient flow, revenue, and overall success. As each practice is trained in these areas, participants can test new ideas in their office and evaluate their success. Employers want to ensure a positive outcome of their investment in the practice.

The consultant believes that each staff member has his or her unique responsibilities, which results in the practice operating more efficiently as each person masters his or her own position. These responsibilities bring accountability to each person for his or her job performance. As consultant introduces specific systems that address different sections or departments of the practice, and the dental team is requested to incorporate them into their every operation. These systems assist in reducing paperwork while providing ways to backtrack when a task is not performed in the most optimal manner. The incorporation of computers and software programs has altered many applications performed in the dental office, and it is becoming increasingly necessary for dental professionals to have technical knowledge and skill. Some of these systems will be discussed later when exploring the duties of staff and the dental hygienist in a clinical setting.

One of the most common drawbacks, as seen by dentists, dental hygienists, and staff members attending management training seminars, is that all of the systems designed and promoted by a particular consultant do not fit the organizational or operating structure of the practice. This may be due to the demographic composition of the patients, the numbers of patients seen each day, the specialty of the practice, or numerous other reasons. Sometimes, the dentist and the staff decide not to incorporate a particular system because they feel it will not benefit the overall production of the practice. A particular system may complicate a task rather than make it easier and more streamlined.

As a result, most dental practices choose to customize their offices by selecting the systems they feel will work more easily and efficiently. A system customized according to the needs of the staff and the practice will more likely be successful and used by all team members. Staff compliance is also likely to be higher. Overall, by selecting systems that best fit the practice, an increase in efficiency and **production** (the amount and cost of services provided to patients per day, week, month, or year) is ensured. When the dental practice operates effectively as a business, patients receive quality care and education by all those who have participated in making their working environment successful.

MANAGEMENT STYLES

As dental hygienists begin a new career, they may find themselves working in more than one dental office. Typically, most dental hygienists choose to work part-time, which may be two to three days per week. Consequently, each office will operate differently from the next, and each will expect the dental hygienist to fall in line with the philosophy of the team and the practice. Leadership in each office may also be unique. Most employees assume that the employer or the dentist is the authority figure and is responsible for making all decisions having to do with the practice and its operations. This is not true for all practices, however. One may find that many employers leave the managing to the receptionist, who may double as the office manager. Some practices will have a receptionist and an office manager, while others are truly managed by the dentist. Additionally, not all managers actually work in the office. Some dental and dental hygiene practices may hire an outside firm to complete all business transactions, such as paying the office bills, billing dental insurance claims, employee payroll, and receivables collections. Thus, the manager may be located elsewhere and seen in the office only when he or she picks up necessary materials.

Leadership styles will also range in the practices you have chosen to work with. The first style is identified as **authoritative management.** This is when the dentist makes all the decisions necessary during the daily operations of the practice. Auxiliaries carry out the specific requests or orders of the employer. This management style does not allow for staff members to take part in any decisions that may affect them or the duties they must carry out in performing their specific jobs within the practice. Additionally, it does not allow for staff members to feel as though they are a part of a team. The dentist in this role may seek to hire employees who are passive in nature so as to avoid any potential conflict in decisions. Authoritative management does not allow for open communication or exchange of ideas that could possibly lead to increased production for the practice and increased patient dental care. Dental hygienists who display confidence and assertiveness may find they are not suited to this type of working environment.

Free-rein management is when there does not seem to be anyone in the management position. In fact, many times employees may describe the practice as operating in a chaotic environment, as ideas and decisions change on a daily basis. There is no consistency or united direction for the practice. The dentist may appear to have a very relaxed personality and working style, while more than one staff member displays dominant characteristics and leadership. Organization is relatively nonexistent because the dentist and staff have not established short-term or long-term goals for the business. Dental hygienists may find that communication and effectiveness is lacking in this type of environment due to lack of interest by the dentist and staff to develop specific channels. This system works for them; thus they see no reason for change. Those who possess high organizational skills may find that they are unable to work effectively in a free-rein environment.

The third category of management styles is **participatory management.** As the term implies, all staff members are a part of the decision-making process. This tends to be advantageous not only for the dentist, dental hygienist, and the staff, but for the patients as well. Just as management consultants feel that each staff member is valuable in his or her contribution to the practice, so too does participatory management. Each staff member shares responsibility for the decisions and the treatment of patients. Open communication is encouraged and free-flowing ideas can be exchanged. The employer's objectives are shared by all members in order for the business to be successful. This results in a better working environment for staff, as they are contributing to the longevity of their careers while working toward a common goal.

THE TEAM CONCEPT

As previously mentioned, management consultants identified the need to incorporate the entire dental staff to assist in meeting the goals of the dentist and his or her practice. This would take teamwork. Each staff member responsible for accomplishing his or her daily duties had to also be knowledgeable about the duties of all other staff members. Thus, the **team concept** was developed.

What does the team consist of? The dentist, dental hygienist, dental assistant, office manager, receptionist, insurance coordinator, and dental laboratory technician are all team members.

Dentists are licensed professionals whose main goal is to improve oral health and provide restorative care. This may include any endodontic therapy and periodontal therapy. Dentists may also specialize in certain aspects of dentistry, such as periodontics or orthodontics; however, the majority of dentists are general practitioners who provide numerous treatment procedures.

Dental hygienists are also licensed professionals who have undergone extensive education that enables them to perform preventive care and patient education. Dental assistants can also be licensed professionals. Some states provide a certificate (CDA) and some states provide a registered (RDA) status. When a dental assistant is certified or registered, he or she is able to perform expanded functions within the scope of his or her state's dental practice regulations. Usually, any licensed practitioner will be required to attend continuing education courses in order to maintain a license. Whatever the education or license, each person has certain obligations to the consumer as well as duties within the position they hold.

Additionally, the office will employ an office manager, a receptionist, an insurance coordinator, and sometimes a dental laboratory technician. Each of these positions will have specific duties designed by the practice.

As you can see, each office will have personnel for the business, or "front office," whose duties are separate from those of the assistant or dental hygienist working with patients and the dentist in operatories, or the "back office." However, the front office team cannot perform its duties efficiently unless the team working in the back office presents accurate patient information and treatment. Once this information is received, patient billing and insurance claims can be effectively accomplished daily. The same holds true for the dentist, dental assistants, and dental hygienists. The front office team is responsible for scheduling patients and their treatment efficiently to ensure that those in the back office performing treatment procedures can do so without being overworked or running behind schedule. Again, open communication and understanding by team members of the various aspects of the dental practice will provide for a low-stress, highly productive practice.

Defining Staff Roles

Each practice that dental hygienists are associated with will likely vary in size and scope of services. Many practices have adopted a mission statement. Mission statements are designed to provide philosophical direction to the employees and outline expectations to meet stated goals, as well as to guarantee quality care to patients. The scope and goals of the practice are what the employer uses to assist in his or her decision for hiring the number of staff members that are required for the practice to carry out procedures efficiently. When a practice does not hire enough employees, the existing staff is overworked and many tasks may be left undone and eventually forgotten. In such circumstances, quality assurance cannot be guaranteed to the consumer. In offices where there may be an excess number of employees, the employer may find that increased socializing takes place. Patients may get ignored while staff is under the impression that "someone else" is taking care of them. Employees get bored waiting for something to do, and many may not possess the self-motivation to stay busy. Both of these scenarios result in decreased office production and financial loss.

As mentioned, the goals of the practice often influence the number of office personnel, dental assistants, and dental hygienists to be hired so as to meet those goals outlined by the employer. Most practices will have **policy manuals** that describe the duties of each employee's position. Policy manuals will be discussed in depth later in Chapter 10, "Seeking the Dental Hygiene Position." It is essential for team members to understand what is expected of them during their association with the practice, as this eliminates confusion about what their job description entails. Each state has specific duties outlined in its dental practice act that describes allowable duties for licensed professionals. All licensed professionals should be aware of the legal duties allowed within their scope of practice. Defining each employee's role will assist in maintaining a smoothly operating practice for the dentist and a better working environment for team members.

CROSSTRAINING

When the employer brings in management consultants, **crosstraining** is encouraged for all team members. This means that each member in the office will be able to perform the duties of another position in the event of illness or long-term absences, thus eliminating the need to hire a new employee or someone on a temporary basis. Crosstraining helps maintain the harmony of the office and the efficiency of the business, and patients' treatment can be provided more efficiently as well. The limitation of crosstraining lies with *licensed* professionals. For example, the front office receptionist is not able to perform any duties of the certified or registered dental assistant or dental hygienist. However, he or she may be able to assist in procedures that do not require licensed education and training, such as seating and dismissing patients or helping to set up or break down operatories.

Furthermore, the dental assistant or dental hygienist may often be asked to perform some front office procedures, such as computer entries, filing, or insurance billing. Dental practices that incorporate such crosstraining techniques are able to run more smoothly whenever unforeseen circumstances arise. Do not be surprised when asked to perform such other functions as a part of the team.

STAFF MEETINGS AND THEIR BENEFITS

Consulting firms and business consultants advocate regular staff meetings for dental offices. As a team member, everyone has the responsibility to contribute to improving the daily operations of the business. The frequency and scope of staff meetings will be at the discretion of the employer and his or her team. Many offices find that a monthly meeting is sufficient to exchange information and present new ideas for consideration or implementation. Other offices find they require a weekly meeting. A number of topics may be discussed in staff meetings. Many employers prefer to share the financial portion of the practice so that all employees are aware of what it takes to operate as a business. Many times, employees become so involved with providing health care that they forget that the practice is a small business within the community. The staff also has the opportunity to share in the concerns and successes of the business. Open communication plays an important role in the success of not only the business, but of those who participate in the team.

Another popular meeting style is the morning **huddle.** Many dental offices that have already gone through a professional practice management program have incorporated morning huddles. During huddles, team members convene 15 to 30 minutes prior to the onset of their day to discuss pertinent information about scheduled patients and the treatment to be performed. They may also look at logistics or plan for certain dental assistants to handle certain cases. Huddles also allow the team to prepare possible difficult cases as well as set aside time for emergency calls. Additionally, the dentist and the dental hygienist will go over patient information so that both understand what may be expected for each individual case. The morning huddle is beneficial to all team members and sets the stage for a smooth and productive day. It also allows for the staff to identify operational strengths and weaknesses on a daily basis.

Staff meetings, in general, allow all employees to provide valuable information that will benefit each individual and the team collectively. Some topics that may be included for staff meetings are

- Developing a mission statement for the practice.
- Developing office policy where all members are comfortable.

- Understanding the quality and standard of care the practice desires to deliver.
- Understanding the business of oral health care delivery.
- Setting of financial goals for the practice.
- Generating and implementing a staff recognition or bonus plan.
- Reviewing the daily schedule for changes.

All of these topics are imperative to the dental practice as a business in order to achieve its goals and realize success.

Each team member is essential to specific duties to the practice and the care it provides to its patients. Differences will be found in every practice. Dental hygienists will also find that their goals and objectives change and become more focused with increased clinical experience and through interacting with different practices and management styles.

Although dental hygiene and dentistry go hand-in-hand for providing complete oral health care to consumers, as a licensed professional, the new dental hygiene graduate will find that the discipline of dental hygiene can be a diverse and rewarding experience.

EXPECTATIONS AND PUBLIC RELATIONS

Employers' Expectations

Although the dental hygienist's main task is providing preventive services, the ability to market all services offered to consumers by the practice will be essential in terms of the practice being a small business. As patients become members of a practice, the image represented to them by staff members assists in augmenting the success of the practice.

From the employer's perspective, he or she understands the foundation of dental hygiene education and training. Dental hygienists are hired by practices to provide the care they have been taught to provide. In addition to the foundation of dental hygiene care and treatment, there are two key factors in a practice that underlie the clinical aspect: **public relations** and **marketing.** These factors are rarely discussed between employers and employees unless the business has gone through management training and has learned to employ these aspects to enhance its business. The practice is there to serve the public. However, the public may not return if the staff as a whole does not represent the employer and themselves in a positive manner. Patients see the dental hygienist and the staff as representatives of the practice, as does the employer. Appearance, demeanor, and skills are indicative of the overall personality of the business.

Public relations deal with image. Public relations require a variety of programs designed to promote and protect a company's image or its individual products (Kotler, 1997). As part of a dental team and a practice, this is one way of being part of a program that must promote itself and its services to remain a viable business. The dental hygienist's ability to represent himself or herself as a team member and a skilled preventive care specialist is of interest to the employer and management because image is how the general public relates to the practice. The role of the dental hygienist becomes important as many patients see them as the experts for preventive oral health care and products designed to improve and maintain oral health. When beginning to provide oral health care, the dental hygienist is likely to see a patient only once in the first six months of employment. That first impression represents not only the practice, but also the employer's ability to select the most compatible person for the business. Thus public relations and image become an important part of the dental hygiene profession. The astute dental hygienist will use public relations to enhance patient relationships, which can assist in improved understanding of the dental hygiene profession among consumers.

As you gain experience and become more acquainted with the patients, you find out some of the concerns they have with dental hygienists. The more common concerns, or complaints, are that dental hygienists are too rough and that they often run behind schedule. Personalities do not always mesh between the dental hygienist and a patient. Interpersonal skills become intertwined with public relation skills. Both are needed to insure that patients in the practice are comfortable with you as the new professional, and the employer and office management are comfortable that the right decision was made to add you to their team. Some of the skills that will be required to enhance public relations are communication, patience, and empathy.

Communication skills are essential. Being able to express ideas and recommendations to patients in a confident and positive manner will enhance their compliance and respect for your professionalism. Many clinicians tend to speak to patients in a demeaning tone or to sound as though they are reprimanding them. Negative communication will not be as effective as positive communication skills. Speak to patients as though they were friends or relatives. As the saying goes, treat others as you would want to be treated.

Have patience with your patients. When dental hygienists first begin their career, many may feel as though they should be making gigantic strides toward improved oral health among their patients. This does not always happen, and in fact it could take years before some patients change their habits. Empathy and understanding of each individual will enhance your professional personality and augment your public relations skills.

The general public does not always understand how important oral health care is and how it affects total body health, or how important dental hygiene education, skills, and career are to the new practitioner. In order to promote the profession and elevate public opinion, dental hygienists find themselves explaining the education and credentials they have for performing the procedures required. This, of course, is a good thing. It creates ease among the patients treated, while increasing their understanding and knowledge of dental hygienists and the dental hygiene profession.

With the rising interest in decreasing dental hygiene education by increasing **preceptorship** training (training received on the job), it is an advantage for the licensed dental hygienist to also educate patients about the dental hygiene profession. Fine-tuning public relations skills that enhance the overall image of the practice and the professional may help to bridge the gap in the general public's perception.

Public relations can involve many aspects of personality, education, and professionalism. As dental hygienists become more comfortable with their new careers, public relation skills will increase to include a broad spectrum of topics. These skills will assist in elevating public opinion of the practice with which the dental hygienist is associated as well as of dental hygiene profession.

Your Expectations

Just as potential employers have expectations, so will new graduates when they begin to discuss the duties required in each practice. During dental hygiene education, and for those who are new to the dental field, it may be an advantage to observe a practicing dental hygienist during regular office hours. This may enhance the overall picture of what really goes on in the practice and of a standard schedule for dental hygiene. Another way to gather information on what a practice expects from a dental hygienist is to seek a mentor in the community where you plan to practice after licensure or in the community where the dental hygiene program is located.

Keep in mind that clinical practice is only one aspect of the dental hygiene career. Recall the six roles of the dental hygienist. If you have dental hygiene contacts in other areas, such as in corporate positions, education, or public service, spend some time with those professionals to learn about the numerous options for dental hygiene positions. Spending some time with a seasoned professional in any career setting will allow you to obtain a more comprehensive picture of what occurs when settled into this new career.

Expectations of Staff

Staff or team members may perceive that new members are similar to themselves. They may expect the new member to automatically fall into place and know exactly where things are stored and located in the office. Established staff members often forget how disoriented new employees are when it comes to finding supplies and equipment.

For the office manager and front office staff, expectations may be similar to the employers' expectations. They may expect that the dental hygienist will be open to making phone calls and confirming appointments or filing patient charts if there is down time. The office may be under the assumption that the dental hygienist is willing to assist in ordering supplies and putting them away as they are received. As a team member, it is important to remember that everyone in the practice has the same goal: to work together productively to provide quality dental care. This also may mean that everyone is open to helping out in other departments in order to maintain scheduling demands. These are examples of why you should prepare questions regarding the job description for each interview you choose to pursue. It is important to understand the daily operations of the office and what has been the general operation in the past with former employees and dental hygienists. Decreasing the possibility of first day jitters or mistakes is essential to making a good first impression on new coworkers and the patients seen that first day.

Expectations of Patients

Being the new person is one part of employment that many people can relate to. Patients of an established practice can be savvy to new faces, high staff turnover, as well as negative atmospheres in the office. The dental office is not everyone's favorite place to visit, although many professionals find this difficult to understand.

Patients expect that the dental staff, whether new or not, are experienced in all aspects of treatment procedures, materials, equipment, and operations. There is a period of adjustment in every new position. The dental hygienist must learn the location of materials and supplies while learning the equipment. He or she must also learn charting systems, computer systems, and appointment policies, and may also need to become familiar with how services are charged and billed to insurance companies. Practitioners who are replacing a person who just retired from the practice will want to orient patients to themselves and their dental hygiene philosophy. For some patients, change may not be easy, and their comfort becomes important. This is essential in initiating a new professional relationship. Most often, the new dental hygienist will inform patients that he or she is new to the office and still learning the location and operations of many things in the practice. This information helps the patient understand, for instance, if the practitioner takes more time than usual to complete a procedure or if he or she must stop to ask coworkers for assistance. The more information given to the patient, the more at ease both parties will be during this important first impression. Coworkers and patients are there to assist in the orientation to a new environment; however, be open to learning how the practice operates.

As mentioned, public relations deal with image. How the public, the dental community, and the patients view the practice, the staff, and the practitioners is important to maintaining the longevity and reputation of the practice. This requires building skills for public relations. Interpersonal skills will contribute greatly toward the image of the dental hygienist and the practice.

MARKETING AND THE DENTAL PRACTICE

Marketing is defined as a social and managerial process by which individuals and groups obtain what they need and want through creating, offering, and exchanging products of value with others (Kotler, 1997). Those who seek care in a dental office are fulfilling a need: dental care. Marketing also targets human wants and demands. Wants are desires for specific items that will satisfy the need. Demands are wants for specific products. This means the practice must use marketing techniques to offer their product and services. Marketing is one of the keys to maintaining a successful practice. Marketing includes planning and management. Often, in larger practices a marketing and business manager may be employed to coordinate the many factors of the marketing plan chosen by the employer. For example, it could be the most advanced materials used for restorative procedures or the latest technology for diagnostic and assessment procedures, such as intraoral cameras and digital radiology. Thus, there is an exchange of goods or products to meet the needs of both the practice and the patient; consumers exchange money for services and procedures performed by the dentist, dental hygienist, and staff. So how does marketing relate to the dental hygienist?

Recall the dental materials course during dental hygiene education. During that education, students learned properties of materials and techniques for restorative procedures. Patients who frequent the practice and have regular dental hygiene visits are apt to question the dental hygienist on the latest technology or seek advice on the best and latest dental care products. Addressing these questions for the consumer is how the practice *markets* its services.

Not only the dental hygienist, but also other staff members answer patient inquiries. All staff should be knowledgeable about their specific areas of expertise and should know who in the practice can provide answers to questions they are unsure of. The dentist is likely to contribute to continuing education for licensed employees by including them in courses that promote the latest materials or technology. For licensed professionals, there may be requirements by your state to accumulate a certain number of continuing education units per year or license cycle. Dentistry is a science, and science continues to find improvements for numerous human needs. The more information and education the staff members have on materials, procedures, and techniques, the greater the opportunity to expose patients to procedures that may be of interest to them. When patients are satisfied with the service and with the result of their treatment, the practice sees increased production and revenue. Satisfied consumers tend to refer family and friends who may seek the latest techniques and materials for restorative services. Marketing skills of the staff become an essential portion of the practice, and yet another area of practice management that underlies the delivery of quality dental care.

In an article called "The Vital Role of Practice Marketing," Connie Hazel (1998) lists five reasons that a practice should implement marketing techniques:

1. *The market is constantly changing.*
2. *People forget.*
3. *Marketing strengthens identity.*
4. *Marketing helps to retain long-term patients.*
5. *Marketing gives patients and staff motivation.*

Changes in market occur when patients move away as well as when new families move into an area. Marketing will ensure that both long-time residents and newcomers are aware of the dental practice. Insurance companies also cause market changes as they become more restrictive, limiting dental care options for some patients. If the practice stops promoting itself and its services—accommodating, where possible, for changes in insurance programs—it may see a decrease in patient flow and referrals.

Advertising assaults us on a daily basis and in a tremendous way. Radio, television, print advertising, and the Internet are the primary means by which companies get their messages to us, and they send their messages over and over again—because people forget. Businesses must maintain a public presence, usually through advertising, in order to retain clientele.

Many dental offices rely on word-of-mouth to increase their patient base. While word-of-mouth is effective, it is limited in its market reach. Through advertising, a practice can reach thousands of existing and potential patients, strengthening its identity and assuring consumers that it is here to stay.

Retaining long-term patients is as important as attracting new patients to a practice. Patients generally frequent a practice because of the service they receive and the professionalism of the staff. A practice must also remain progressive, keeping up with the latest procedures and technologies, so that patients are assured that they continue to receive the most modern care available. A practice should promote its advanced services in its marketing strategies.

Both patients and staff are motivated by a practice's effective marketing. Working in an office that is well known in a community elevates the staff morale, and patients are reassured that they have chosen a quality practice for their dental care.

Marketing: The Patient's Health Care

As we have discovered, patients seek dental care because of a need. That need comes in different forms. As a dental hygiene student, you may be familiar with Michele Darby and Margaret Walsh. They have identified 11 human needs as they relate to dental hygiene care, which becomes important for you, as a preventive care specialist, as does understanding the exchange of goods (money) and services (treatment):

- Safety—freedom from harm or danger .
- Freedom from pain/stress—exemption from physical and emotional discomforts.
- Wholesome body image—positive mental representation of one's own body.
- Skin and mucous membrane integrity of the head and neck.
- Nutrition—the need for a balanced diet.

- A biologically sound dentition—need for intact teeth and restorations that provide function.
- Conceptualization and problem solving—to grasp ideas and make sound judgments.
- Appreciation and respect—need for acknowledgment and achievements.
- Self-determination and responsibility—need to exercise firmness of purpose about one's self and behavior.
- Territoriality—to possess a prescribed area of space or knowledge.
- Value system—freedom to develop one' own sense of importance (*Darby & Walsh, Abbreviated*).

When patients seek dental care, they are attempting to fulfill one or a combination of needs. A marketing strategy is able to target specific services that fulfill these needs for consumers. All staff members are expected to be knowledgeable in the materials and techniques that are on the cutting edge of dental care, as this area is also of interest to many patients. These are only a few reasons for maintaining licensure with continuing education courses.

For the dental hygienist, patient needs assist in designing treatment and home care programs for maintaining quality dental hygiene care. Patients want integrity and compassion from their caregiver. Patients want to be assured that they are receiving the best their dollar can buy. Possessing competent marketing skills will help in their assurance.

Marketing the Practice

Dentistry and dental hygiene care has changed dramatically over the past 25 years. There was a time when patient treatment focused on "fixing" whatever ailment the patient complained of. Prevention was not the basis of oral care. Since then, patient care has changed, and the delivery aspect of that care has seen a dramatic transformation.

Dental practices need a positive patient base and **cash flow** to maintain existence in the business world. In order to accomplish this, the practice may focus on creating a niche or may target a particular market that helps them stand out as a leader in dental services within the community. In order to accomplish this task, the business may opt to convert its delivery systems to include those of the latest technology. Technology may include modern equipment, computer programs, and digital radiology. These things can result in higher patient volume and perhaps increased patient referral.

The practice must analyze what they currently offer in the way of programs, which could draw more consumers. After identifying their strengths and weaknesses, the practice can then rely on staff members to market the best programs directly to the patients. Offering them the service that will fulfill their need—the reason they sought service in the first place—is the first and easiest step when patients are physically in the office.

Marketing the practice takes a lot of energy and planning. Many employers will seek professional consultants to focus on the direction the practice or staff may want to pursue. For example, many offices have opted to focus on cosmetic dentistry. Others find they do better at providing family, implant, or other specialty services. Finding a specific niche in the oral health care field means the practice must target its own talents. Marketing dental hygiene means the practice and the dental hygienist must target patient education on the profession and the professional and its important role in total systemic health. Marketing aids the employer, the staff, and the practice in focusing on specific programs that have been chosen to provide to its patients. The overall outcome will result in a profitable business. For those interested in independent practice, refer to Appendix E, "Components of a Marketing Plan."

Marketing Yourself

Along with public relations and the image the dental hygienist presents to the employer, staff, and patients, new practitioners will also become adept in marketing for the practice, techniques, materials, services, and of course themselves. Yes, many do have to market themselves every day. The patients need to know that the dental hygienist is a professional oral care specialist. As mentioned, many patients see their dental prophylaxis as just a cleaning. Most often, dental hygienists encounter patients who are unaware of what this procedure involves, let alone of procedures like root planing. Additionally, they are unaware that it has taken at least four years to get through a dental hygiene education. Even with two-year dental hygiene programs, there have been a number of years for prerequisite education. Consumers are unaware of the spectrum of dental hygiene knowledge. They are unaware of what it takes to maintain a license through continuing education.

These are reasons why marketing becomes an important aspect of dental hygiene. Patients need to understand that the person providing these services is in tune to the latest techniques and materials. Because of continuing education, the dental hygienist will have the ability to provide information patients are seeking. Ultimately, dental hygienists are marketing themselves and all the knowledge acquired over many years. Everything learned is applied to everyday working environments. Patient inquiries require marketing skills that allow the dental hygienist to be the professional consumers want and employers seek.

Marketing Strategies

Other strategies that may be advantageous to the practice and the dental hygienist as a professional will include programs and activities that can bring attention to the practice and help shape it as a leader in the community. Following are some examples that can be used to increase exposure for the office:

1. Become sponsors for local events or organizations, such as children's sports teams, soccer, baseball, and swimming teams. It might also include sponsoring local health fairs and school events.
2. Contribute oral health articles to the local newspaper.
3. Appear on the local television or radio stations to promote National Dental Hygiene Month or other nationally and locally recognized days.
4. Participate in presenting continuing education courses designed for colleagues as well as other health care providers (e.g., nurses aids, nurses, home health aids).

As a member of one's own professional organization, volunteering becomes second nature in promoting oral health.

Marketing and Profit Centers

Profit centers, or mini-profit centers, are another way for the practice to increase its productivity. Profit centers consist of specific products that are offered to patients from within the office. As discussed, it will require continuous marketing to retain existing patients and to acquire new ones. In today's modern dental practice, it can be easy to implement a profit center that not only results in revenue over and above standard dental procedures, but also allows for increased compliance among the patients and may set the practice apart from others in the community. There are advantages and disadvantages of profit centers and possible ethical and legal aspects that may need to be addressed by the practice's business manager and accountant.

As the dental hygienist, your interest lies in getting patients to comply with the recommendations you have prescribed for them so that they maintain better oral health. Most profit centers focus on patient needs and compliance. The most popular patient need (or rather, demand) is teeth whitening or bleaching. This is an easy avenue for the practice to offer a procedure that falls in the latest technology category, fulfills the need (or desire) of the patient, and results in additional income for the practice. Therefore, the practice can set up displays that promote teeth whitening. For example, it may use before and after photos of their patients. Additionally, the practice may have its entire staff whiten their teeth. Now the staff is able to describe the procedure to the interested patient from first-hand experience.

As mentioned for patient compliance, the practice typically finds it can easily focus on products that are recommended by the dental hygienist. These products may be oral irrigation devices, electric toothbrushes, or dentifrices. These products are easily acquired by the office from the manufacturer and offered to the patient for purchase. Many times, the key marketing tool is the convenience. Dental hygienists often recommend certain products due to their **efficacy** or patient acceptance. Patients are apt to purchase the recommended product because it is conveniently located in the office. This too creates additional income for the practice.

Other profit centers include halitosis clinics and products and soft tissue management programs. Halitosis clinics address patients with chronic bad breath. During oral hygiene education courses, students learn that bad breath usually results from bacteria and periodontal disease. However, there are many other reasons, some of which include medications, systemic diseases, and reasons that dentists and professionals cannot diagnose. As a result of this increasing patient need, halitosis clinics have opened throughout the country. The office can purchase specialized equipment and products known as volatile sulfur compounds specifically developed for causes of halitosis. Once the diagnosis is made, patient compliance will be higher when the product can be purchased in the office. Here again is an example of addressing a patient need while marketing a unique service that makes the office stand out from other practices.

Soft tissue management programs are another specialized area for profit centers. These programs are based on the patient's need to improve oral health due to periodontal diseases and pocket depth. Weekly visits are required for dental hygiene treatment as well as patient education and modification. Patient education includes mini-classes. For example, the dental hygienist educates the patient on how to manage oral health using an electric toothbrush and other products combined with frequent professional treatments. Many practices today have soft tissue management protocol. As the dental hygienist, you may be expected to participate in or design a program.

Disadvantages for profit centers may include ethical and moral issues, not to mention legal issues. Ethically, is the practice allowing autonomy? By making certain products available to patients, is the business allowing them to make the choice that is best for them? The practice cannot afford to bring in every type of product on the market. Therefore, it selects certain products based on sales and marketing by the manufacturer. Does this limit the consumer's decision? Should the consumer be allowed to see all products before purchasing a specific model or item? The moral aspect is twofold. The practice believes it is providing a convenience to its patients, yet it is making a profit based on sales. What is the true motivation for including a profit center? As professionals, most dental hygienists prefer not to "sell" dentistry or dental hygiene. The questions are not easily answered, and the dental hygienist will want to feel comfortable and confident that the reasons for a particular profit center fall in line with his or her professional philosophy. Legally, the practice needs to be sure that revenues from sales items are taxed appropriately, if required by state or federal regulations for retail sales. This will require consultation with a tax consultant.

Profit centers are increasing in today's dental office, and it is one way to keep the patient healthy while making the practice unique. The dental hygienist can be an integral part in creating profit centers that address patient needs. Public relations and marketing both play a role in making the practice you work in profitable and successful in the eyes of the consumer. Being a part of the dental hygiene profession will bring a variety of aspects to your new career, increasing the spectrum of knowledge you bring to your patients every day.

SUMMARY

Although the dental practice provides dental care, it is also a small business and must realize a profit to remain a viable source of income for all those who are employed by the practice. The 1980s saw a surge of consultants and consulting firms targeting the dental practice. Many consultants have succeeded in incorporating systems that streamline the daily tasks performed in the dental office. However, not all systems fit easily into every dental practice. Usually, the dentist and his or her team customize the systems to be incorporated. Dental hygienists are typically employed in more than one dental office. Management styles will vary in each practice setting. Authoritative management indicates that the dentist is the decision maker. This does not allow for other staff members to present ideas that may benefit the practice and their working environment. Free-rein management may mean the office operates in a chaotic state, as the authority figure or decision maker cannot be identified. Communication channels have not been identified, as the staff has not seen the need to design such channels. Participatory management implies participation from every staff or team member in the office. Each individual takes an important role in the development of the working environment and the success of the practice. Communication lines remain open and encourage the exchange of ideas.

Defining staff roles decreases potential confusion as to who is responsible for certain tasks in the office. Most practices have developed policy manuals to achieve complete understanding of each staff member's roles. Management consultants advocate crosstraining, as this will maintain smooth operations during staff illnesses or long-term absences. After the dental practice undergoes management training with a professional consulting firm, staff meetings or huddles may be incorporated at intervals determined by the dentist and his or her team members. Implementing regular meetings encourages the team members to plan their day so that it runs smoothly. In addition to daily planning, exchanging ideas for practice development may enhance the overall goals and objectives for the business.

Public relations and marketing are two aspects of the dental practice that underlie meeting the needs and demands of the general public. Public relations deal with the image of the practice, the dentist, and its staff members. Employers rely on staff members to represent and promote the practice to patients as they are treated in the office. This promotes the word of mouth advertising needed to remain a viable community business. Staff members market technology, procedures, and materials to patients. Those who frequent the practice are seeking to fulfill a need or demand. Marketing deals with the exchange of products to fulfill a need. Marketing the ability of the practice to meet those needs is what the employer expects. Continuing education helps to keep the staff members current on the latest trends in dentistry and dental hygiene procedures.

Marketing targets specific human needs. Human needs have been identified as they relate to dental hygiene. Other reasons for marketing are that people move, people forget, and marketing can help retain long-term patients.

Profit centers are a way to increase practice revenue while increasing patient compliance. The dental hygienist can be instrumental in creating a profit center, using products and home care appliances recommended to patients. Profit centers targeting tooth whitening, halitosis, and home care products are more popular and widely accepted by patients.

SELF-TEST

1. Identify the management style in a practice in which you are familiar. Is this style successful for the practice? If not, what style would you recommend, and why?

2. Briefly explain why not all systems recommended by a management consultant may work in every practice.

3. Explain the purpose of the team concept and why this is an advantage.

4. List some topics that may be included during staff meetings or morning huddles. How does this influence the interaction between team members?

5. Identify some of the expectations that were discussed in a past interview and some of the expectations that were not discussed, yet were realized after beginning the job.

6. Using a local telephone book, look at some of the advertisements for dental offices in your area. Identify terms used in the advertisement that promote the *image* of the practice.

7. If you were asked to set up a mini-profit center, what type would you select, why, and how would you set it up? Be as detailed as possible.

CHAPTER 8

The Business of Dental Hygiene

OBJECTIVES

Upon reading the material in this chapter, you will be able to

1. Describe the scope of the *dental hygiene diagnosis.*
2. Discuss *business* aspects for dental hygiene.
3. Discuss *time management* issues and plan a treatment hour.
4. Compare *alternative practice* settings for dental hygienists.

INTRODUCTION

Diagnosing for dental hygienists has become known as the "D-word" for most practitioners. Most states' dental practice regulations specify that the dentist is the only person legally able to diagnose patients' conditions. Although this may be legally accurate, the dental hygienist has a legal, ethical, and moral obligation to diagnose the oral hygiene condition of patients seen every day. Recall the core values beneficence and nonmaleficence discussed in Chapter 2, "Ethical Principles and Core Values." Both terms relate to benefiting the patient. The patient in turn trusts your professional expertise and judgment. *Webster's New World Dictionary* defines *diagnosis* as "the act or process of deciding the nature of a diseased condition by examination of the symptoms." It is a careful examination and analysis of the facts in an attempt to understand or explain something. Dentists diagnose dental disease in general, such as carious lesions and their extent, in order to determine causes and recommend treatment that will remedy the condition. The main concerns for dentists are treating the symptoms, preventing new and recurrent caries, and reconstruction of lost dentition. Why should diagnosis be different for the dental hygienist evaluating the condition of patients' oral hygiene? As you learned during your dental hygiene education and applied in your clinical training, the **dental hygiene diagnosis** serves a completely different purpose than the dental diagnosis. It focuses on problems or potential problems related to oral health and disease versus dental disease (Darby & Walsh, 1995). Licensed dental hygienists are responsible for identifying the deficient human need as related to dental hygiene. Identifying a possible etiology and designing and planning treatment in order to remedy the patient's condition is the goal of each practitioner. As a professional, you will also have to deal with patients' perceptions, beliefs, and attitudes, which requires interpersonal skills and obtaining factual information. Other factors must also be considered if professional services are to be successful. These factors may include:

- *Recognizing the causes (etiology) that resulted in poor oral health.*
- *Identifying the human need the patient is seeking to fulfill.*
- *Patient assessment, such as medical and dental histories.*
- *Recognizing abilities or inabilities of the patient to comply with your recommendations.*
- *Prioritizing dental hygiene treatment, recare, and maintenance.*

Assessment, diagnosis, evaluation, implementation, and interpretation are intertwined when it comes to helping patients fulfill a need. Ethically, licensed practitioners are required to utilize these skills to determine oral health deficits and provide the best treatment. For example, patients are typically eager and expect the dental hygienist to provide them with interpretative results of radiographs. Yet, legally, the dental hygienist cannot diagnose dental disease. However, recall the human needs as related to dental hygiene identified by Darby and Walsh. Using that information, the clinician is now able to identify the human deficit as it relates to the patient's oral hygiene, which is the need for sound dentition. Therefore, after evaluating new radiographs and observing a carious lesion, the dentist can be informed prior to his or her oral examination. Why? Because the patient's need for sound dentition has been identified as the deficit. Generally and legally, final dental diagnosis is always confirmed by the dentist.

The process for the dental hygiene diagnosis includes other factors worthy of discussion. As defined, examination of symptoms and analysis of facts are required before finalizing results. The astute dental hygienist will gather the appropriate data using the medical and dental history along with current information provided by the patient. Using this information, clinicians are able to look for patterns or a series of patterns that assist in developing possible etiologies for the patient's current oral health. Diagnosis takes quality evaluative skills and application of the knowledge gained in dental hygiene school as well as information from continuing education courses. Licensed practitioners will want to continuously build and perfect these skills as they gain experience in the clinical setting. In doing so, the chance of misevaluation will decrease and patients benefit from the clinician's expertise.

Another immediate resource of expertise is the employer. The dentist must also attend continuing education courses and be available for consultation. Working as a team, the staff can ensure that patients in the practice receive quality dental health care.

In dental hygiene education, students may have learned to use terminology that does not specifically lead to diagnosing dental disease: *suspicious*, *signs of*, or *area of concern*. These terms and phrases do not designate dental diagnosis or dental hygiene diagnosis; they simply assist the professional with informing the patient of his or her present condition.

Another example of dental hygiene diagnosis is the clinical evaluation of existing restorations. Upon evaluating patients' restorations, a margin that is faulty and possibly causing recurrent decay may be identified. This would meet the criteria for needing sound dentition and restorations that function. So what is the dental hygienist's responsibility? Using the process for the dental hygiene diagnosis, the practitioner can determine that restorations will need to be replaced. The dentist and the patient will discuss the best dental treatment option; however, as the dental hygienist, you can inform your patient that a defect in the existing restoration is present and treatment may be required.

Using diagnostic skills, dental hygienists focus on problem areas. The basis of preventive treatment is being able to determine the etiology behind current oral hygiene conditions so that modifications are implemented. Patient compliance is an area the clinician targets when evaluating for the most effective home care recommendations. Patients often complain that their dental hygienist reprimands them every time they have a dental prophylaxis. Can you imagine what it might be like if the patient sees a new dental hygienist who is unfamiliar with his or her oral health history? During dental hygiene education, make an effort to look for the positive aspects in patients and the successes they have achieved. Look for strengths in patients and take advantage of them when discussing home care. Everyone wants to be praised for his or her accomplishments. Otherwise, no one would attempt to make improvements. Patients want to be treated by someone who sees their strengths, not their weaknesses. Interpersonal skills become imperative when discussing these aspects of oral health.

Examples such as these display what is involved in the diagnosis process. Ethically, the clinician must determine the oral health deficit and inform patients. The dental hygiene diagnosis assists the preventive care specialist to present accurate information to the patient so that the patient has the opportunity to participate in his or her oral health care. It is a valuable tool for the dental hygienist. Use it for processing patient information prior to designing a treatment plan, recare, and maintenance. Each patient is an individual and each dental hygiene diagnosis and treatment plan is customized to that individual's needs. The dental hygiene field is unique and rewarding for many who choose this career. Each patient, each case, and each dental hygienist is unique and should be viewed and treated with that uniqueness in mind.

MAXIMIZING SKILLS

Now that public relations and marketing skills have been identified and defined, the dental hygienist must be able to recognize his or her own limits. New graduates may be hesitant to realize at the start of their new career that they are unable to perform the required treatment on cases they have just planned. Those with experience realize their limits and skills and know that a specialist will better serve their patient. Participating as a team member, professional resources are available: the employer and the professional community he or she has developed while providing patient services. Dental hygienists will also have many of these resources at their disposal.

Numerous aspects become incorporated into the development of a dental hygiene professional. For example, most dental hygienists obtained at least four years of formal education. Many have been exposed to the scientific background of dental hygiene theory, practice, dental materials, and technology. Some have gained knowledge about public relations, marketing, and interpersonal communication. And of course, each will continuously be exposed to educational courses that are applicable to his or her licensure and interests. How does this apply to each dental hygienist and his or her patient?

By using expert resources and specialists, preventive care specialists are better serving the overall health of patients. This expansion of expertise allows each to exercise critical thinking and evaluative skills. Recall the meaning of beneficence: doing what will benefit or help a person or patient. Maximizing your clinical and intellectual skills will insure doing the best you can for patients.

THE BUSINESS OF DENTAL HYGIENE

Profitability in the dental hygiene department is one important factor many employers frequently review. There are those employers who believe that dental hygiene loses revenue, while many others believe dental hygiene increases revenue for the office. However, those employers may not realize the revenue that is referred back to them by their dental hygienists when faulty restorations or new carious lesions have been identified during the patients semiannual prophylaxis, not to mention the numerous patients who are seeking cosmetic improvements with their dentition and smile. Instead, they may see only the outgoing salary and possible benefits the dental hygienist "costs" the practice.

Dental practices may view their hygiene department as just that, a department. This means that **overhead** costs need to be considered and monitored, as well as the amount of production the dental hygienist can produce given daily, weekly, and monthly scheduled procedures. What can a dental hygienist produce? Recall the meaning of production: the total cost of procedures performed over a given period of time. Table 8–1 gives an example of what a typical day might entail, based on a variety of dental hygiene services on a sample day with eight 1-hour appointments.

The results for the day show revenue of $1,085. As a student, this kind of day appears overwhelming, especially since many have had 3-hour to 4-hour clinic sessions during their program. However, as dental hygienists enter the working environment, this may be a schedule that finds them within the first 30 days of their career.

Now that revenue has been explained, the cost of doing dental hygiene business requires equal time. The costs of utilities such as electric, water, and gas are not discussed here, because this model uses the dental hygienist as an employee within a practice. Utilities would be used by the

Table 8–1 Dental Hygiene Production

Qty.	Procedure	Fee	Production
5	Adult prophylaxis treatments	$ 65	$325
2	Root planing/quadrants	150	300
1	Child prophylaxis treatment w/fluoride	45	45
4	Bitewing radiographs	50	200
1	Full set radiographs	95	95
4	Sealants	30	120
		TOTAL	**$ 1,085**

employer also, and would be used in calculating overhead for the practice as a whole. For dental hygienists that seek or enter independent practice, utilities would need to be included and also calculated in total costs. So, how does overhead affect dental hygiene? Mainly, it has to do with the oral hygiene aids given to each patient and with the salary of the dental hygienist. If the dental hygienist receives benefits, this too would be an expense for the employer. Using the sample day from Table 8–2 itemizes approximate daily expenses.

Table 8–2 Approximate Daily Expenses for a Dental Hygiene Day

	Oral Health Aids & Procedures	Cost to Practice
8 patients =	8 toothbrushes @ $2.00	$16.00
	8 floss dispensers @ .25	2.00
	2 interdental brushes @ $1.00	2.00
	8 toothpaste tubes @ $1.00	8.00
	Total	**$28.00**
If radiographs are included:		
	4 BWX @ $2.00	$8.00
	1 FMX @ $9.00	9.00
Sealant Material	4 @ $1.00	4.00
	Total	**$21.00**
DH Salary	$32/hour × 8	$256.00
Benefits (if applicable @ 10% of salary)		$25.60
TOTAL EXPENSES FOR THE DAY		**$320.60**
Profit received by the practice $ 1,085 − 332.60		**$752.40**

As shown, the practice will receive a profit for a day that may include all of the represented procedures. Profit for dental hygiene procedures will not be as large as dental procedures. The cost for a quadrant of root planing is far from the cost of a crown or 3-unit bridge. In addition, this sample does not take into account patients who cancel or fail their appointment at the last minute. It also does not take into account insurance payments received. Thus, profit will fluctuate on a daily basis. What may not fluctuate is the salary and benefit package paid to the dental hygienist, unless the compensation is based on percentage of production (to be explained in Chapter 10, "Seeking the Dental Hygiene Position"). Although there are numerous factors that are seen daily in the dental practice, a profit is likely to be realized.

DENTAL INSURANCE AND HYGIENE SERVICES

Fees for dental hygiene services vary throughout the country. In addition, dental insurance coverage varies greatly, depending on the type of insurance consumers carry, and many consumers have no dental insurance coverage. Payment for dental and dental hygiene services will also vary, anywhere from zero to 100 percent. Insurance companies will also vary their payment depending on the type of hygiene services provided to the consumer. For example, a regular prophylaxis may be covered and paid at 100 percent, where quadrant root planing may be covered and paid at 50 to 70 percent. Again, it depends on what type of dental coverage the consumer holds.

Although there are a number of insurance plans available to the consumer, those described here are among the most common found in dental practices, both private and public. Private-pay patients are those who do not have insurance and will pay for services rendered out-of-pocket. These patients will pay the **usual customary and reasonable** (UCR) fees that have been determined by the dentist in the practice with which they are associated. Most dental corporations use UCR. UCR fees can be found in all dental practices and will typically be submitted to insurance companies, which assist in maintaining the level of fees in a particular geographic area. For example, if Practice A charges $70 per dental prophylaxis, Practice B may not be able to charge $90 for the same service if located in the same city or county. Thus, the consumer benefits from this type of regulation and will not feel overcharged for the same basic service. **Preferred Provider Organization** (PPO) coverage contracts with dental practices to provide dental services to the consumer. The amount of payment to the practice or dentist is set in a fee schedule determined by the insurance company. **Health maintenance organizations** (HMO) and **dental health maintenance organizations** (DHMO) are other types of insurance coverage where the consumer may be limited to dental care within the organization, which may include their own dental facilities. They have accepted responsibility and financial risks for providing dental services. HMOs and DHMOs may also be limited to providing coverage to consumers within a specific geographic area and perhaps a specified time period. Payments to the dentists again tend to be based on a specific scale or percentage based on UCR fees but determined by the insurance company. **State assistance** for medical and dental coverage is another way for low-income families (especially children) to receive needed oral health care. Each state has guidelines and qualifications, and there may be a limited number of dental practices offering to incorporate this kind of dental coverage into their practice. Many communities will provide community health and dental facilities to those in this category. Students may become familiar with these families or these facilities during their community oral health course. PPO, HMO, and DHMO coverage are major factors for managed care. **Capitation** systems are based on the fact that the dentist, not a third party, takes the risk for delivering dental care. The dentist is compensated a fixed fee based on the number of patients enrolled in this system rather than on the type of services rendered. Incorporating these types of clientele in a dental practice requires business savvy and advanced scheduling skills in order for the practice to realize an acceptable profit.

The type of insurance held will determine billing procedures for patients with insurance coverage. Some insurance companies may require their own dental billing form. Others may accept a universal form that can be used for numerous insurance companies. State plans may have a specific form designed to meet their specific needs. Additionally, there may be requirements for **preauthorizing** planned treatment. This means that once the dental hygienist has determined how to approach a patient's treatment, the insurance company may require prior authorization. For example, if the patient has been determined to need quadrant therapy in order to return to better oral health, the insurance company may request a copy of the radiographs and the periodontal charting in order to confirm that quadrant therapy is warranted. For the insurance company, this is a way to monitor the expenses paid for services as well as to monitor the treatment received by the patient. Most insurance companies will not provide benefits if the treatment is over assessed. Additionally, most insurance companies will place a limit on how often procedures can be performed. For example, periodontal treatment may be allowed only once every three years.

There are insurance companies and dental coverage that do not require pre-authorization for treatment. Each insurance plan, much like each patient, will need to be viewed independently. As the oral health provider, the dental hygienist will want to be familiar with the insurance processes that are required from the practice. The length of the learning curve will vary for each practitioner. Those who are familiar with dental insurance will assimilate to the protocol sooner than those who have entered the dental hygiene field for the first time. Table 8–3 gives examples of some of the insurance codes that are pertinent to dental hygiene treatment. It will be an advantage for the dental hygienist to become familiar with these codes so that patient's treatment and insurance coverage are maximized.

Although Table 8–3 represents only a portion of insurance codes that are used in the dental office, this will help the dental hygienist in understanding what is available when planning treatment. It should be mentioned at this point that despite the fact that many patients will have some kind of insurance benefits, not all procedures are within their particular plan. For example, notice the code 01310, nutritional counseling. Even though this code is included in all UCR fees and recognized by dental insurance companies, many plans do not pay benefits for patients to receive this treatment. Therefore, it is wise to review what may or may not be covered in the patient's insurance plan with the office manager or insurance coordinator, as they may have a better understanding of how the insurance company handles these types of services.

How various insurance coverages and managed care plans affect the overall income and profitability of the practice is an area too extensive for the scope of this text. For those who seek positions in facilities that accept many of these programs, expanded information will be readily available to assist in the comprehension of how these programs operate on a daily basis.

CONTINUING CARE AND RECALL SYSTEMS

During any dental hygiene education, students become very familiar with continuing care or recall systems. In order to assist patients in maintaining oral health, the dental hygienist wants to see them periodically. This means the patient is recalled at certain intervals. A continuing care system is integral to continued patient flow in the practice and can be seen as the lifeline to long-term success. Although most often patients will receive an

Table 8–3   Insurance Codes and Nomenclature for Dental Hygiene Related Procedures Abbreviated

00100-00999 I. Diagnostic

Clinical and Oral Evaluation

00120 Periodic oral evaluation

00140 Limited oral evaluation - problem focused

00150 Comprehensive oral evaluation

00160 Detailed and extensive oral evaluation-problem focused, by report

Radiographs

00210 Intraoral—complete series (including bitewings)

00220 Intraoral—periapical; first film

00230 Intraoral—periapical; each additional film

00240 Intraoral—occlusal film

00270 Bitewings—single film

00272 Bitewings—two films

00274 Bitewings—four films

00330 Panoramic film

Tests and Laboratory Examinations

00415 Bacteriologic studies for determination of pathologic agents

00425 Caries susceptibility tests

00460 Pulp vitality tests

00470 Diagnostic casts

00471 Diagnostic photographs

00501 Histopathologic examinations

00502 Other oral pathology procedures, by report

00999 Unspecified diagnostic procedure, by report

II. Preventive

Dental Prophylaxis

01110 Prophylaxis—adult

01120 Prophylaxis—child

(continued)

Table 8–3 Insurance Codes and Nomenclature for Dental
Hygiene Related Procedures Abbreviated (*continued*)

II. Preventive (*continued*)

01201 Topical application of fluoride (including prophylaxis)/child

01203 Topical application of fluoride (prophylaxis not included)/child

01204 Topical application of fluoride (prophylaxis not included)/adult

01205 Topical application of fluoride (including prophylaxis)/adult

01310 Nutritional counseling for the control of dental disease

01320 Tobacco counseling for the control and prevention of disease

01330 Oral hygiene instructions

01351 Sealant—per tooth

04000-04999 V. Periodontics/Surgical Procedures

Adjunctive periodontal surgery

04220 Gingival curettage

04341 Periodontal scaling and root planing-per quadrant

04355 Full mouth debridement to enable comprehensive periodontal evaluation
and diagnosis

04381 Localized delivery of chemotherapeutic agents via controlled release vehicle into diseased crevicular tissue, per tooth, by report

04910 Periodontal maintenance procedures (following active therapy)

04920 Unscheduled dressing change

04999 Unspecified periodontal procedure, by report

Miscellaneous Services

09910 Application of desensitizing medicaments

09920 Behavior management, by report

09999 Unspecified adjunctive procedure, by report

oral prophylaxis and examination, many will also be seen for various other reasons, some of which apply to post-dental treatment: extractions, orthodontic treatment, and follow-up visits after endodontic therapy.

Extensive research and knowledge of the cause and effect of periodontal health and its effect on systemic health recognizes that patient education is more important than ever if the dental hygienist and the patient are to be successful in oral health care. Successful systems will incorporate several factors: oral health education, motivation, consistent follow-up, and appropriate treatment.

Continuing care systems are varied, and each practice will use the system that best suits its needs for managing patients. The **advanced appointment system** is increasingly becoming the most widely used in many areas. As each patient completes a dental hygiene visit, he or she is scheduled for the next visit prior to leaving the office. By scheduling in advance, the patient has committed that day and time to the dental hygienist. The disadvantages are that many patients do not know their work or personal schedules that far in advance. Additionally, the dentist and the dental hygienist cannot predict they will not be ill on the day the patient has scheduled. A **mail system** consists of mailing a card to the patients during the month they are due for their regular appointment. This system places the responsibility on the patient, as he or she will need to call and schedule the appointment. The disadvantage is that the patient may forget to call or may ignore the notice. Currently, with so many computer systems and software programs, most practices are able to enter recall due dates as the patient leaves. Later, a report can be printed showing the last date of services, types of services received, the specific interval recommended by the dental hygienist, and the date of the patient's next appointment.

In creating an effective hygiene department, the dental hygienist can identify objectives that the continuing care system should address. These objectives could include

1. customizing the approach to treatment.
2. encouraging patient compliance and return for future appointments.
3. obtaining a commitment from the patient to accept treatment recommendations.
4. motivating patients to take an active role in their oral health and treatment.
5. educating patients on the significance of continuing care and its value relative to restorative treatment.

In addition to establishing workable and attainable objectives, the dental hygiene department may decide to incorporate a philosophy that all participants can apply to their every day working routine. It is imperative for each practitioner in the department to establish and document the diagnosis as it pertains to the patient's current oral health condition. Each patient should be informed of the diagnosis and counseled as to the recommended treatment and any options that apply. Finally, treatment will be provided by the professional as indicated by the diagnosis and discussed with the patient.

Developing an effective hygiene department may be a challenge for those who are asked to participate. Many factors need to be considered. Therefore, planning plays a significant role during initiation stages. Continuous review of the philosophy and objectives will be required by all participants to best maintain smooth operations.

TIME MANAGEMENT

For a new graduate, time management is the most common concern. Most programs may have allowed students three to four hours for each clinic session. Now, on day one of a new job, the dental hygienist has been cut down to one hour for each patient. Additionally, he or she is expected to see an average of eight patients that day and to stay on schedule. After all, the patients are not new to the practice. They anticipate the same appointment they usually attend at each recall visit. You, as the new employee and new dental hygienist, are the newest addition to the practice.

Many practices allow the dental hygienist 60-minute appointments. However, this is not always the case. Some offices allow 45-minute or 50-minute appointments. The procedures performed by the clinician will be identical regardless of what time allowance is given per appointment. As a result, the new practitioner must plan the hour or time allotted in a manner so that all patients can be seen on time. Time management is an issue that many employers are aware of, and many are willing to work with you as you gain experience in the office. One of the dental assistants may be assigned to the dental hygienist as he or she becomes familiar with the equipment, location of materials, and schedule. Thus, do not hesitate in discussing this aspect of the new position during interviews.

How can time management be addressed when beginning a new position? One area to consider is radiographs. Discuss the possibility of having one of the dental assistants take radiographs that may be required for those scheduled with the dental hygienist. This will allow extra time in that hour for clinical needs such as periodontal charting or scaling. Other suggestions may arise during discussion of time management with potential employers.

For those who obtain employment in practices that accept PPO, HMO, or state assistance plans, the time allotment for dental hygiene appointments could be much shorter. Recall that managed care programs require special scheduling in order for the practice to break even or realize a profit. This leads to 45-minute and sometimes even 30-minute appointments. Again, the dental hygienist is expected to provide normal hygiene services regardless of the time allowed. Many new practitioners are unable to work within these time constraints. Most often, the new practitioner has difficulty feeling as though he or she is benefiting the patient. This can result in ethical dilemmas or distress. Ethical obligations for dental hygienists for patients are at the forefront of every procedure performed. Thus, when interviewing for dental hygiene positions that include managed care programs, be sure to discuss the time allowed for procedures, and be sure that you are ethically and morally comfortable that the patient is receiving the best care available.

Time management will improve quickly for each new practitioner. Open communication with the dental assistant and employer will assist in making the transition smoother while increasing efficiency with each appointment.

WORKING WITH OTHER DENTAL HYGIENISTS

When entering a new position, be sure to ask the same questions as for any interview. During dental hygiene school, most students purchase their own instruments. When working in one or more practice, the employer may supply the instruments; however, more than one clinician will be sharing the same sets. This may become problematic, since each clinician sharpens and scales differently. Several options can be employed to alleviate problems with instruments when shared. The employer may decide to purchase instruments for each hygienist; thus each will have several sets to last an entire day. Another option is for the dental hygienist to purchase his or her own instruments. If the dental hygienist is employed in one office, the instruments can be stored in the operatory. If employed in two or more practices, the dental hygienist may choose to travel with his or her instruments.

Some practices provide the dental hygienist with a dental assistant. This may be a rare convenience for many seasoned practitioners, yet there are practices that incorporate this aspect. Sometimes, the employer provides a dental assistant only during the transition period of the new association with the practice. Dental assistants assigned to the dental hygienists will perform adjunct duties such as taking radiographs, setting up instrument trays, sterilization procedures, seating patients, and numerous other activities. This arrangement will allow for increased production by the hygiene department, less stress among the clinicians, and efficient appointments for the patients.

ALTERNATIVE PRACTICE SETTINGS/INDEPENDENT PRACTICE

When students graduate and begin their career, many will find themselves in a private practice setting. The majority of dentists have chosen to own and operate their own practice, whether it is in general dentistry or in one of the dental specialties. However, dental hygiene services are needed in other settings. The dental hygienist can work in elementary school settings, nonprofit community dental facilities, hospitals, military bases, as well as places like federal Indian reservations. Currently, there is a movement toward access to care for all individuals. In 2000, the US Surgeon General's Report addressed the oral health of America for the first time (US Department of Health and Human Services, 2000). This report brought forward the reality of access to care needed by millions, many of whom are children. Organized dentistry, dental hygiene, and many other health organizations are working to make improvements in this area. Increasing access for consumers provides not only emergency care but much needed preventive care. These settings can be rewarding for all that participate, including consumers. When given the opportunity to work in an alternative setting, the new graduate is encouraged to explore the option. Seek more information on how the dental hygiene professional can assist in providing care for those who cannot be treated in a traditional dental office environment.

Independent practice began its appearance as early as 1976. Linda Krol, a California dental hygienist, was the first to own and manage her own practice. Since then several states have attempted and continue efforts in this direction. For the dental hygiene profession, this is seen as another avenue for access to care for many who cannot find their way into a traditional dental practice. Colorado successfully passed legislation allowing independent practice for dental hygienists. Restrictions still applied to root planing and radiograph procedures. These services are scheduled by dental hygienists in a dental practice they may be associated with.

In 1986, California began a Health Manpower Pilot Project (HMPP #139) designed to study the safety of and access to dental hygiene services in unsupervised settings. Success was realized in 1999 with the licensure for the Registered Dental Hygienist in Alternative Practice (RDHAP). Today, there are 16 dental hygienists who own and operate their own dental hygiene business. Some are freestanding offices, while other choose to use mobile equipment and provide services in nursing care or residential care facilities.

The state of Washington also has some independent practices that operate similarly to those in California. In New Mexico, dental hygienists are practicing in what is termed a "collaborative practice" based on criteria that has been established by a committee and state governing board. This includes allowing the dental hygienist to provide education, assessment, preventive, therapeutic, and clinical services without supervision. They too can work in a variety of settings: schools, nursing facilities, and private dental hygiene practice. This movement is a future pathway for the dental hygienist as a professional. It is designed to provide services to those who are underserved for a variety of reasons. As members of the professional organization, each will have the opportunity to influence the direction of his or her new career.

SUMMARY

The dental hygiene diagnosis is separate from the dental diagnosis. Analysis of factual information provided by patients and determining the human deficit present is required for the dental hygienist to develop the appropriate diagnosis for patients' current oral health conditions. Eleven human needs have been identified in relation to dental hygiene, and the astute dental hygienist will be able to use these needs to inform patients of their oral health requirements. Additionally, the dental hygienist must deal with the beliefs, attitudes, and perceptions of their patients, which will require effective communication skills to insure patient compliance.

Dental hygienists typically focus on problem areas rather than on areas in the patients' mouths that may be showing signs of health. Many patients complain that the dental hygienist reprimands them. Turning the approach toward the positive will allow the dental hygienist to use the strengths of their patients rather than point out the weaknesses. Patients want to be recognized for their accomplishments; thus refocusing on their achievements may prove beneficial in maintaining patient compliance.

When employed in private practice, each practitioner has the opportunity to use experts and specialists associated with the employer and the practice.

Maximizing your skills as a professional dental hygienist includes understanding your total background as well as acquired information learned on a daily basis. Formal education, continuing education, and education from interactions with employers, coworkers, and patients contribute to your professional composition. Everyone benefits when these skills are used to their greatest potential.

SELF-TEST

1. Describe the differences between the dental diagnosis and the dental hygiene diagnosis.
2. Develop several scenarios for a dental hygiene schedule and calculate production and expenses. What is the resulting profit for the practice?
3. Using Table 8–3, identify the insurance codes that would be used for four quadrants of root planing, a full set of radiographs, and a periodontal maintenance visit.
4. Given one hour for a dental hygiene visit, list the procedures needed to be performed on a patient who has come in for a six-month prophylaxis. The procedures should also include periodontal charting, radiographs, and an examination by the dentist. Using this list, determine how much time will be needed for each procedure in order to stay within the 60-minute time period.
   a. What would be the time needed for the same procedures, given a 45-minute appointment?
   b. How about a 30-minute appointment? Can you identify areas that will suffer when the time becomes too short?
5. Using Appendix E, what might one need to consider and plan if selecting to enter independent practice? Select two of the items on the checklist and develop an action plan that you could implement. (Hint: Create a step-by-step plan)

CASE STUDY

Contributed by Debi Gerger, RDH, BS, MPH, Program/Clinic Coordinator, San Joaquin Valley College, Rancho Cucamonga, CA.

Given the following information, develop a dental hygiene diagnosis. Identify the deficient human need, and design a treatment plan with referral if required.

As a new licentiate, you interview for a dental hygiene position in a "caring and thorough" general practice. The office manager describes the benefits to include an above average salary, paid holidays and vacations. You accept the position.

On your first day of work, the manager hands you your schedule. You immediately notice a different schedule than what you were told. Now you see that you have 40 minutes per patient instead of the 60 minutes discussed at the interview.

You begin your day with a patient who had his new patient exam and radiographs with the dentist three months ago. After reviewing the medical history, you evaluate the radiographs. There is generalized horizontal bone loss of 2 mm and multiple areas of radiographic calculus. Next, you look at the dentist's treatment plan, which indicates the patient is to receive a scaling and polishing. You begin with a tissue and calculus assessment and taking pocket probing depths that all indicate at *least* early periodontal disease.

In developing your dental hygiene diagnosis, consider the ethical principles of beneficence and nonmaleficence. Recognize that the patient trusts that you are giving him or her the best care. Think about what is meant by informed consent.

Discussion: One of the first items that you should be concerned about is why the patient was diagnosed for what appears to be scaling and polishing. Was it a misdiagnosis because the exam was too quick, not thorough, or because the dentist is ignorant (uninformed) in regards to periodontal assessment and diagnosis? Are the patients receiving substandard care because of insurance reasons such as capitation plans (flat fees received based on patient visits)? Is the office focused on completing patients in one visit, with no exceptions?

The ethical principles of beneficence and nonmaleficence direct us to do what is best for the patient. Is a prophylaxis best for the patient? Is some care better than no care at all?

A dental hygiene diagnosis that would include full data collections to develop a treatment plan of oral hygiene instruction and quadrant root planing is the simple component. The complex component is how to handle patient communication, including informed consent, and how to handle the communication with the dentist. This creates an ethical dilemma that many dental hygienists choose to ignore. What will you do?

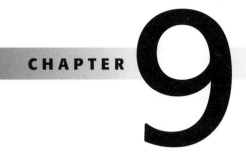

CHAPTER 9

Technology and Dental Hygiene

OBJECTIVES

Upon reading the material in this chapter, you will be able to

1. Discuss the development of computer use in the dental practice.
2. Describe how computer software benefits dental hygiene procedures.
3. Describe advantages and disadvantages for *intraoral cameras*.
4. Identify the differences between standard radiography and *digital radiography*.
5. Identify various *automated periodontal charting systems*.
6. Identify the uses for *laser technology* in dental hygiene.

INTRODUCTION

It seems the majority of modern communications includes aspects of Internet and computer technology. Computers in general have expanded by leaps and bounds, yet come in smaller packages and appear to have no limits. However, the average life span for a computer system, at present, is about three years. Hardware (the equipment) and software (the programs) change so quickly, consumers must purchase computer systems for what they believe their needs will be in the future rather than what their needs are now. Computers vary greatly in their speed and memory capacity, which is high priority when researching what is available to the buyer. Thus various styles can meet various needs. Furthermore, systems that once required an entire room can now be held in the palm of a hand. As computers enter the practice and the operatory, dental professionals must be prepared to change the way they practice. Additionally, consumers must be prepared to change the way they receive oral health care. Consumers have now become co-therapists with their dental hygienist. This means that the patient becomes more active as a participant in how dental hygiene care is delivered. They are able to contribute to the decisions made that will affect their health.

The personal PC was first introduced to the business office to keep track of patient accounts, billing, insurance claims, and the dental services provided each day (production). Prior to their incorporation, office personnel used "peg board" systems (hand written receipts of charges and money collected) and ledger cards to keep track of charges and payments. This meant that the manager or accountant had to balance charges against collections on a daily basis to maintain a balanced book. As computers became more prominent for business tasks, these systems quickly became antiquated. Today, computers can be found in each operatory. The dentist, the dental hygienist, and the assistants have become experts in computer systems and applying the benefits they provide for patient education and motivation. The practitioner, via Internet or CD-ROM applications, can access health and drug information within a few minutes. Oral health care delivery has taken a turn onto the technology expressway such that "personal touch" now has a microchip attached.

The "big boom" for computer systems has skyrocketed within the last 10 years. In 1996, over 400 commercial dental computer systems were available (Neiburger, 1998, p. 96). It is estimated that 80 to 90 percent of U.S. dentists own computers and operate them in their practices (Reis-Schmidt, 1998, p. 26). Smaller and faster computer systems are available to businesses, making this type of technology more cost effective for managing a dental practice. The big question for every practice is which computer system and what type of technology is best for its needs. The purchase of such equipment will require extensive research, as they can be costly to the practice ($10,000 to $20,000). In order for the practice to invest in computer systems, the cost must be justified. Justification comes in several forms, most of which include patient education and motivation, which leads to increased sales of dental services.

The majority of dental programs are similar, although some may be more "user friendly." Ease of use is an aspect to keep in mind when the dental hygienist is required to learn multiple computer systems as a result of having more than one employer. With the numerous tasks performed by the dental hygienist in providing oral health care to patients, why take on additional responsibility for incorporating technology into a dental hygiene appointment? How much technology is too much? Or is there a need for more?

INTRAORAL CAMERAS

One of the first purchases by most dental practices is the intraoral camera. Over 50 percent of dentists are using intraoral camera systems (Reis-Schmidt, 1998, p. 30). As with most technological inventions, the intraoral camera has seen its maturity by way of size, quality, cost, and user friendliness. Intraoral cameras began in the mid 1980s as large hand-held video cameras that somehow were adapted for use in the oral cavity (Wagner, 1995, p. 23). The processor and monitor were not as remote as they can be today. Earlier versions of the intraoral camera had wires and cables that remained connected during use, which meant the operatory became overcrowded with bulky equipment and staff members. Cost of equipment may have been prohibitive for many businesses. Intraoral cameras have now become smaller, with increased picture quality and remote control. Their operations can be learned by all staff members within a day.

Several companies manufacture intraoral cameras. They vary slightly in their applications; however, components will be similar. Each system setup will include a video monitor, a light source (typically halogen), a processor for the camera, the handpiece (camera) with fiber optic cables, a printer, the remote control, and the foot control. When systems are more complex, a video player or other components may be included. Depending on the type of system purchased, the cost ranges from $4,000 to $12,000. Generally, intraoral camera systems can be housed on a mobile cart. This allows the camera to be used in all areas of the practice and by any staff member. Mobile units assist in keeping costs down for the practice. Intraoral cameras can also be installed as stationary systems. This is accomplished by mounting a monitor on a wall in each operatory, and a camera is placed in each room for individual use by the clinician. No one has to share the system. In an effort to continually improve aspects of intraoral systems, the handpieces have become smaller, autoclavable, or used with disposable sleeves. Computer chips are being incorporated to provide improved digital images, and multiple lenses allow clearer pictures and closer views. Photo printers allow the clinician to develop an actual color photo (similar to a Polaroid) of the intraoral images taken by the camera. The practitioner also has the option of capturing the image using the remote control or the foot control. When provided assistance, the dental hygienist can operate the camera for the image desired while the dental assistant captures the image with the remote control (Figure 9–1). If operating the intraoral system alone, the foot control is utilized.

The intraoral systems will typically allow the operator a choice of multiple images on one photo or a single image. How can the dental hygienist use this technology to benefit dental hygiene procedures?

The initial use for intraoral cameras was in educating the patient on needed restorations and assisting the dentist in clinical examinations. The dentist could show the patient where restorations were needed and justify

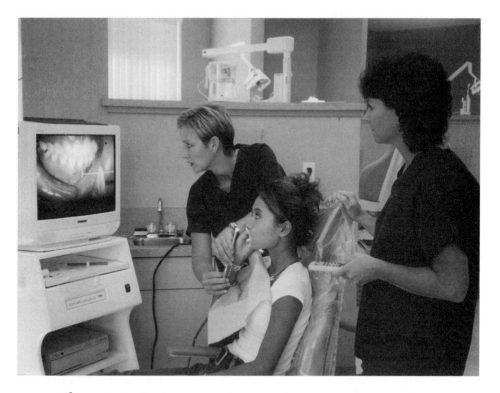

Figure 9–1 Students operating an intraoral camera for patient education.

the recommended procedure. The patient, on the other hand, was able to see exactly what the dentist was observing. It may have been a faulty margin on an existing restoration, fracture lines, or weakened tooth structure. This improved the overall patient-dentist relationship while increasing overall revenue for the practice. As the focus shifted toward improving oral health, the intraoral camera became a partner with the dental hygienist. By incorporating this technology, the dental hygienist is now able to educate and motivate patients to become a co-therapist in their own oral health.

As professionals, we know that the patient must understand exactly why his or her oral condition is important as related to overall health. Systemic diseases are influenced by what occurs in the oral cavity. When the patient can be presented a photo of an area that needs improvement, he or she can better comprehend what the dental hygienist is talking about. As the saying goes, pictures are worth a thousand words. The dental professional now has an invaluable tool, which will assist in improving oral health by way of patient education. Intraoral cameras can now be integrated with computer software to incorporate voice-activated charting systems and digital radiography. Each system is dependent on the software selected by the practice and the level of sophistication desired by the business.

Uses for intraoral cameras in the dental practice and for the dental professional include

- Patient education and motivation
- Patient compliance
- Insurance documentation
- Restoration evaluation
- Changes in soft or hard tissues
- Postoperative evaluation
- Patient cases (before and after processes)
- Diagnostic verification

Disadvantages for the intraoral camera stem from the learning curve it will take for staff members to become adept at maneuvering the camera to capture the image desired. Although most systems and their components are similar, it will take time to fine-tune the hand-eye coordination skills. Another disadvantage is the time it will take from the dental hygiene appointment, especially when the dental hygienist has to incorporate needed or required photos for patient education or postoperative evaluations. However, most professionals who become familiar with intraoral systems will find that their benefits outweigh disadvantages. Thus, it is only a matter of time and practice for the dental hygienists to become familiar with intraoral camera use so their patients realize success in their oral health. For more information on intraoral cameras, visit *www.gendex.com* or enter the keywords *intraoral cameras.*

Tips for Operating the Intraoral Camera

- **Patient positioning** using the camera while the patient is in an upright position will assist in getting the best angle for the area being photographed. Operators standing behind the patient's head will be able to view the monitor to ensure the location of the camera.
- **Stabilizing the camera.** Those who begin using the camera will find that they are unable to keep it steady. Using a fulcrum will help to decrease the instability and blurring of the photograph.
- **Involve the patient.** As mentioned, cameras usually have a remote control. When the dental assistant is unavailable, the patient will be the next best option. This allows him or her to participate in the treatment.
- **Multiple copies.** Be sure to print more than one copy of the photo you are targeting. Patients enjoy seeing the improvement, the insurance company may benefit from this format of documentation, and accurate documentation can be kept in the patient chart.

DIGITAL RADIOGRAPHY

Dental radiography has gone from dip tanks to auto processors to laptop computer screens. Even with the advent of automated processors for radiographs, taking and developing x-rays remains a time consuming task, especially when new patients enter the practice and a full set of radiographs is required. Automated processors decreased the time for development and made it easier to handle chemicals. However, in an effort to continually improve oral health care delivery and patient education, digital radiography technology has been introduced and is fast becoming a selected preference over standard x-ray procedures. Here again, the dental professional has to modify the way procedures and patient assessment are approached. The consumers must also become more educated in how they are receiving treatment and how it affects their overall health.

Instead of opting to expose dental film via radiation, processing, and mounting them prior to clinical examination of the patient, more and more businesses are using digital imaging, which results in faster exposure time, decreased radiation exposure, and immediate viewing of radiographic images. Numerous companies manufacture digital radiography systems, yet the components will be similar in their operations. There are two approaches to digital imaging for dental x-rays. First, sensors can be used that are wired directly to the computer (**direct approach**). Instead of using film and radiation, digital systems use sensors containing a charge-coupled device (CCD). Sensors are rectangular in shape and come in different sizes, similar to x-ray film; however, they are slightly thicker. A remote module transmits data to a computer. Much like an intraoral camera, the computer is able to capture the image transmitted from the sensor to the computer monitor or screen. Once in the computer system, the images can be used for patient education, processing insurance requests, as well as diagnostic purposes. In addition to these uses, the images can be manipulated by colorization, which provides other information that may be diagnostically useful to the dentist or dental hygienist. For information on the direct systems, visit the Web sites of Schick Technologies and Trophy.

The **indirect approach** employs the use of a reusable film-like packet without wires. The "film" is a photo phosphor plate that is activated using x-ray then scanned in special devices that read the image from the plate (Babinski, 1999). A scanner digitizes the image and sends it to the computer. Process time takes about four minutes, but the resolution factor is greater. This system also allows taking panoramic images where the direct systems are limited to single images. The main advantage for indirect systems is that the phosphor plates are thinner. The amount of time to obtain and develop radiographs with this system is about the same as traditional radiographs. The indirect approach is similar to conventional radiography; thus dental personnel may be more comfortable with the format. Students interested in additional research on indirect systems can visit the Web sites of Gendex and Digora.

Most dentists will research these systems to be sure they will meet the needs of the practice, not only for patient education, but to assist in efficient operations. The average cost for digital radiography systems ranges from $9,000 to $12,000 (Emmott, 1999, p. 102). Currently, some mobile systems average over $22,000 (Highlander Dental, 2000).

Table 9–1 compares the advantages and disadvantages of digital radiography. Digital radiography continues to evolve and the dental hygienist will do well to maintain current information on new systems. By doing so,

Table 9-1 Advantages and Disadvantages of Digital Radiography

Advantages	Disadvantages
• Increased speed of development	• Learning curve varies
• Reduced radiation exposure	• Thickness and size of sensors
• Images can be modified/enhanced	• Computer operations
• Increased storage of images	• Sterilization protocol
• Increased efficiency	• Housing additional computer equipment
• Increased resolution	• Setup costs
	• Legal issues
	• Infection control

transitions to new practices become easier and career alternatives present greater opportunities.

LEGAL CONSIDERATIONS

With the increasing popularity of digital radiography, legal considerations are an aspect that all practitioners must be aware of. As with traditional dental radiographs, federal and state laws exist regulating the control and use of x-ray equipment in the United States. Recall that state laws require those who operate radiographic equipment to possess a certificate or license after receiving the proper training and education. Although states vary in their requirements, one of the most important legal considerations for dental radiology is **risk management.** Certain policies and procedures must be followed in order to avoid legal action that a patient may file.

During your study of ethics, you became familiar with *informed consent.* The patient gives consent for treatment after being presented all pertinent information regarding that treatment. And as *autonomy* is applied, each patient has the right to make decisions about his or her health care, even if it means they choose to deny treatment. Additionally, **liability** implies that the dental professional is liable for procedures that are performed in obtaining radiographs and for using that diagnostic tool in informing the patient of his or her current oral condition. Many dental hygienists fail to realize that they are as liable as other certified staff members for radiographic procedures. When lawsuits occur, they are usually malpractice suits, which means any and all licensed or certified professionals can be named in the suit.

Digital radiographs are likely to fall under the same legal guidelines as traditional radiographs when it comes to informed consent and liability protocol. However, since digital radiographs are stored on a disk rather than in a film holder, how long must they be kept on file? Who has ownership of the radiographs on the disk? What happens when the insurance company requests a duplicate to evaluate the need for a restoration? These are but a few of the questions facing those practices that have opted for technology. The legal system has not been able to keep up with the technological advances that include computer systems and information technology. With traditional radiographs, courts have ruled that ownership is retained by the dentist (Johnson, et al., 1999, p. 478). Patients pay for the skill of the professional interpretation to diagnose radiographs. Copies of radiographs are often requested by other practitioners and patients and can be easily supplied. Furthermore, traditional radiographs are required to be retained for seven years by the dentist (p. 479). Yet, when radiographs are stored on a disk, seven years later the software program may not be able to read the disk. Formats for computer programs change quickly, and this is an important legal consideration with such technology. Given the ability to manipulate digital radiographs via colorization techniques, there are questions as to whether they will be considered useful evidence in lawsuits (Haring & Jansen, 2000, p. 393). Film manufacturers are in the process of developing mechanisms that may safeguard original images and allow only copies to be altered. As you can see, there is much to consider in using technology. As a licensed professional, continuous education must occur in order to remain current on trends that may affect dental hygiene care or practice.

COMPUTERIZED PERIODONTAL CHARTING SYSTEMS

Computer systems for diagnosis and treatment have become more common, and numerous software programs are available to the dental profession. Automated probing systems appeared in the late 1980s with the introduction of the INTERPROBE system by Bausch & Lomb. This system used a disposable probe tip that provided periodontal measurements, which printed out on a specific form. The 1980s seem like centuries ago when it comes to technology advancement. The early equipment was bulky and awkward, with foot controls and cords that had to be near the operator. Setting up the equipment and removing it after use was sometimes time consuming. Today's trend is to create smaller, faster, and overall more efficient systems. With voice activation technology, for example, the results of a periodontal record can be charted in the computer as the dental hygienist speaks into a headset, enabling hands-free probing and eliminating the need to search for a dental assistant with a free moment. Better yet, the dental hygienist no longer needs to memorize several numbers then turn, deglove or overglove, and document the numbers on the periodontal chart. The time savings alone can be as much as 75 percent (Wagner, 1995, p. 24). Voice activated systems require fewer equipment parts around the patient and in the operatory, as the computer terminal is the same one used for numerous applications. Many computer manufacturers are working toward advancing improved oral health by incorporating systems that assist the dental professionals in providing the education needed for those they treat. All charting systems (see Figure 9–2 for an example) will include pocket depths, mobility, furcation involvement, recession, and notations for bleeding or suppuration. This makes the periodontal examination detailed and complete.

In the working environment, you will encounter computer systems and diagnostic programs that are new to you, and you will require training to become familiar with their use.

LASERS

As a dental hygiene student, you may have been informed of laser therapy in dental hygiene procedures. Although many programs do not have the time to incorporate laser technology into the curriculum, it is a procedure the dental hygienists can perform with recommended postgraduate training. Lasers are used for several procedures, including tooth whitening and soft tissue curettage. The most common laser used for dental hygiene therapy is the ND-Yag (neodymium:yttrium-aluminum-garnet). Its most popular use is post root planing for deep pockets that tend to harbor bacteria that prevent optimal healing. Therefore, the laser is used to obliterate bacteria, allowing improved healing. It is highly recommended that the operator acquire training to become certified in its operations and use. The disadvantage of laser use is that longevity of its effects typically end after about 60 days. Reevaluation of the laser-treated site may indicate additional treatment is needed.

Laser use for tooth-whitening procedures is demonstrated by placing a mixture of bleaching paste on the tooth. A rubber dam protects gingival tissues. The argon or CO_2 lasers are used for this process. The laser light is then directed at the tooth surface to activate the whitening process. The results are obvious, but may last only about six months. Dental hygien-

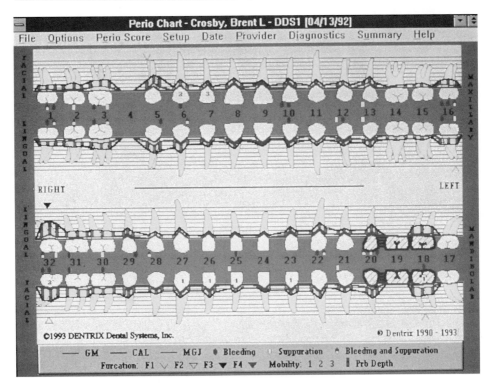

Figure 9–2 Samples of Dentrix clinical and periodontal charts (© 2000 Dentrix Dental Systems, Inc.).

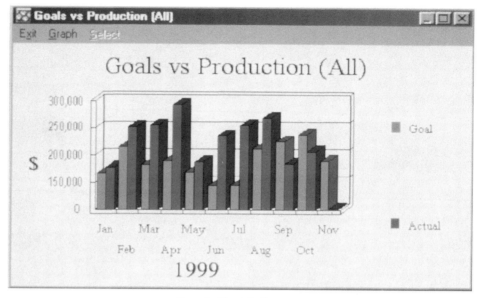

Sample Dentrix Reports

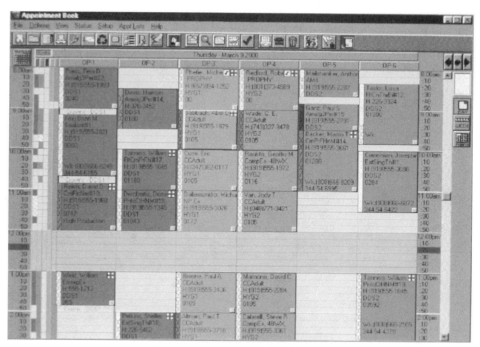

Dentrix Appointment Scheduler

Figure 9–2   *Continued*

ists' use of laser in this format may differ from state to state. It is best to understand the legal regulations in the state that you practice. Furthermore, at present, the use of lasers for periodontal surgery is not supported by research and is therefore discouraged. The use of lasers for other periodontal purposes, such as subgingival curettage, is equally unsubstantiated and is also not recommended (Carranza, 1996, p. 591). However, according to Bob Dalton of American Dental Technologies, laser curettage may likely become the number one application for soft tissue lasers as oral health care treatment expands. Dalton points out that there has been a shift from caries to periodontal disease. Lasers can be expensive, ranging from $17,000 to $24, 000.

In October 1998, the Food and Drug Administration (FDA) approved the use of a laser for caries removal and Class I, II, and V preparation. This laser is offered by Biolase Technology and uses temperature-controlled, high-speed atomized water droplets to cut hard tissue.

PAIN-FREE INJECTIONS

A computer-controlled local anesthesia delivery system, the Wand, delivers anesthetic solution using precise pressure and volume rations (flow-rate). The standard cartridges are used and are placed onto the tabletop unit. There is no metal syringe, but a soft vinyl disposable handpiece with a needle attached. The operator holds the handpiece much like a pen. This technique can be used for all types of injections. Visually, this is less intimidating to the patient. The Wand has been used in clinical practice since 1995. The basic operation for the Wand (shown in Figure 9–3) is as follows:

1. A standard anesthetic cartridge is placed into the holder and twisted into place.
2. The disposable handpiece and needle are positioned at the insertion site.
3. The needle is then inserted, and the solution is delivered via foot control at a slow rate controlled by the computer unit.

COSMETIC IMAGING AND IN-OFFICE FABRICATION OF RESTORATIONS

Several years ago computer-aided systems were introduced into the practice to help the dentist in porcelain restorations. It was a time-saving factor for the patient, as the restoration could be completed in one visit.

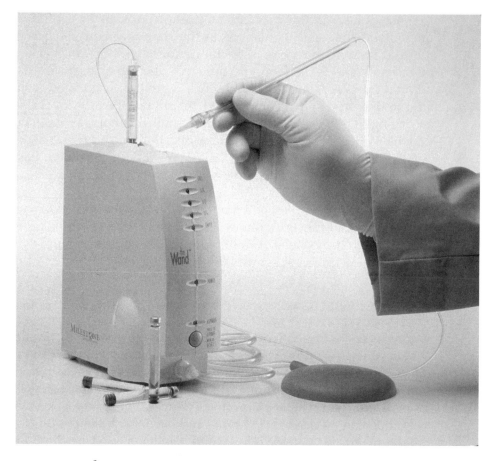

Figure 9–3 The Wand, offered by Milestone Scientific.

Upon the system's initial introduction, many restorations were not as successful as hoped, due to the materials used and patient sensitivity.

Since that time, better systems have appeared and are beginning to reenter the practice. These systems are known as CAD/CAM or computer-aided design, computer-aided manufacturing. These systems are designed to view the restorative impression (the negative) in a three-dimensional state, then produce the ceramic restoration based on the image produced by the computer. These systems produce only ceramic restorations. The second-generation systems seem to be more user friendly and to manufacture improved final products. Aesthetics are improved as well, as is longevity of the restoration itself. Several companies offer these second-generation systems: Patterson Dental, Nobel, and Nobel AB (Masek, 1999, p. 66).

Computers are also being used to generate the results of contemplated cosmetic procedures. TigerImage is software that has been developed to provide such an image to patients who are seeking aesthetic changes. This system is economical, as the patient is allowed to view the results prior to investing in a treatment that he or she may not like. TigerImage can provide the patient with images of elimination of diastemas, tooth lengthening, repair of fractures, crowns, veneers, and full-mouth cosmetic improvements. TigerImage is offered by Televere Systems, *www.televere.com* (DPR, 1999). This is only one software package available to the dental professional. As technology improves, these systems as well as computerized restorative options become an integral part of providing total oral health care.

CHARTLESS PATIENT RECORDS

Since the introduction of computer systems to manage patient records and the evolution into the operatory to include periodontal records and radiographs, many practices are opting to transcend from paper documents to computer records. With computer systems, the copyrights and ownership of software is designated to the inventor or manufacturer. It is considered intellectual property. However, regarding the creation of electronic patient records, the property is another legal situation that may not have been addressed in every state as of yet. Additionally, those who choose to maintain all patient records on the computer are taking a risk in the event that the computer "crashes" and all information is lost. The advantage still lies with paper documents, as the legal system recognizes this as standard. Computer storage of patient information requires extensive research and planning. Consider this: The information taken today using the programs available to businesses may not be readable by the software programs used 10 years from now. This is a major consideration for practices that choose to rid themselves of paper documents.

As a dental hygienist working in a practice where chartless organization has become the norm, consider inquiring about the legal aspects of electronic patient records especially if requested by the patient, another dental practice, or the insurance company. Somehow the information must be transferable, and likely a hard copy (paper document) is printed and provided to those requesting information. As a health professional, be aware of what trends may affect dental hygiene practice and the practitioner.

DOES PATIENT CARE SUFFER?

Given all this technology to enhance the delivery of oral health care, does the patient care suffer? Have we, as professionals, lost that personal touch to computer analysis? For decades patients have been accustomed to sympathy, empathy, and nurturing guidance that assists in patient education, motivation, and compliance. With computers in the operatories or equipment being rolled into the room prior to any treatment, many dental hygienists are taking the time to ensure that each patient still feels that personal touch in some manner. Verbal communication, compassion, and eye contact remain viable segments of maintaining interpersonal skills. Patients must know that their dental professional still cares about them as a whole person. Thus, regardless of intraoral cameras, automated periodontal systems, and paperless patient records, every dental hygienist has the opportunity to enhance interpersonal communication and skills that are vital to all humans.

HOW TECHNOLOGY BENEFITS DENTAL HYGIENE

Although computers may be intimidating for some, technology as a whole assists the dental hygienist in many aspects of total patient care. Intraoral cameras have the capacity to validate the dental hygiene diagnosis made by the clinician. Patients are able to see the areas discussed and the need for improvement or the result of periodontal therapy. Images displayed on the video monitor help to confirm what the practitioner is attempting to convey to the patient. Digital radiology may decrease the amount of time x-ray processing takes and will also allow the patient to follow the practitioner while evaluating x-rays. An initial learning curve is inevitable, but the fact that the radiographs can be altered for specific information can be an advantage to the dental hygienist.

Laser use varies in dental hygiene therapy. Post graduate courses are required prior to its use by a dental hygienist. Automated periodontal charting systems and computers in the operatory are likely to be the area that increases in overall use by the dental hygienist. This technology can improve time and patient management. As there are many software programs available at present, and likely to be more in the future, the dental hygienist should remain current on technology that will affect how preventive services are administered.

Other Technology Options

As technology continues to enter the office and as dental hygienists begin to incorporate more technology into patient care, other pieces of equipment may be found in the practice.

- Digital cameras record photos that are kept on disk and entered into the computer.
- Digital panoramic x-rays.
- Cosmetic imaging uses the computer and special software to provide patients a visual image of how cosmetic restorations may enhance their appearance (Victor Dental).
- Computerized occlusal analysis systems allow the patient to bite on a sensor, which will provide a color-coded contour image of the occlusal surface. This also allows dentists to record the balance of the patient's bite and center of force (T-scan II).

Summary

Computers have entered the dental practice by way of practice management and patient assessment. Software and hardware come in a variety of packages and are manufactured by numerous companies. Each practice will select the system that best suits its needs. Intraoral cameras were among the first equipment to be introduced into the dental practice. Initially, it was viewed as a mechanism to increase production, but has become an integral part of patient education. Although lasers have been used for specific procedures in patient treatment, this area may see greater improvement and use as technology continues to become more user friendly. Advanced certification courses are available to licensed dental hygienists interested in adding this skill.

Digital radiography is quickly becoming incorporated into the average dental practice. It allows the practice to make an investment in technology while eliminating the need to have developing chemicals and processors on hand. Most radiography systems are easily learned. The main advantages include decreased processing time and the ability to manipulate the images for patient education and comprehension of recommended treatment.

Automated periodontal systems may see a higher use and acceptance among the dental hygiene community. Some of these systems allow hands-free operation, which improves time management and decreases the need for assistance in recording the information. Patients become educated as the practitioner calls the probing results into a microphone, documenting the information in the computer.

SELF-TEST

1. Provide a brief history of the introduction of computers to dentistry in general.
2. List three uses for intraoral cameras by the dental hygienist and how they would be incorporated into the dental hygiene appointment.
3. What are disadvantages of intraoral cameras?
4. Compare and contrast the differences in digital radiography systems.
5. List the advantages and disadvantages of digital radiography.
6. Describe how automated periodontal charting systems assist the dental hygienist.
7. List some of the uses for lasers. How are they incorporated into dental hygiene therapy?

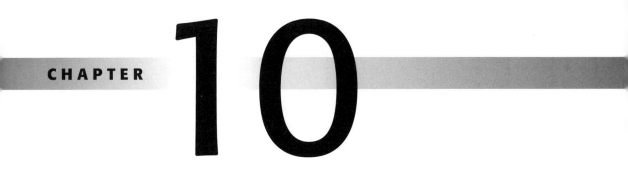

Seeking the Dental Hygiene Position

OBJECTIVES

Upon reading the material in this chapter, you will be able to

1. Recognize the scope of *job searching.*
2. Identify different *employment opportunities* for dental hygienists.
3. Discuss the *process of interviews* between employers and employees.
4. Identify the advantages and disadvantages of *working interviews.*
5. Identify contents and needs for office *policy manuals.*
6. Discuss *benefits* as they relate to the dental hygienist.
7. Apply *negotiating skills* related to employee benefits.

INTRODUCTION

Upon graduation, dental hygienists begin to look at what it will to take to find the right position. Many students relocate from their home community to attend dental hygiene school. Thus, they may decide to stay in their new location or return home to begin their career. Searching for a job after graduation requires some research and planning. The new graduates should investigate open positions within their community, the surrounding communities, and practices that have difficulty getting dental hygienists to consider their offer.

Whether the educational program you attended is located in an urban or rural area, you need to look at several factors that may help to determine where to begin practice. One major consideration includes available dental hygiene positions.

Surveys done by the American Dental Association (ADA) indicate that there is a shortage of dental hygienists in certain parts of the country. This may be partially true, since there are areas where dental hygienists do not reside. However, employment surveys conducted by the American Dental Hygienists' Association (ADHA) indicate that a maldistribution of dental hygienists may be more accurate. This means that dental hygienists may be plentiful in urban communities, while rural areas experience a lack of clinicians to provide dental hygiene services. This may be a result of dental hygienists being unwilling to relocate or commute to surrounding areas.

Another possible reason for lack of open positions may stem from dental hygienists choosing to stay in permanent positions within their communities. As learned, dental hygiene can be a very flexible career. Many will have the opportunity to work as much or as little as they like. Additionally, many practitioners are satisfied with their positions and their employers; thus shifting in dental hygiene positions will not happen frequently. Should this occur in the area where you reside, relocation to a community where dental hygiene positions are more abundant may be the next best alternative. Many dental hygienists are unable to relocate, however, due to family ties and commitments, but commuting is an option to consider.

A 30-minute drive one-way to work can be a long distance for some, while for others, commuting means at least 45 to 60 minutes or more. Regardless of the distance, the time it takes to commute to work is another factor to consider when searching for a position. Commuting to outlying communities is another opportunity to gain employment more quickly if relocation is not an option.

Overnight stays may decrease the expense of the commute, wear and tear on the vehicle, as well as fuel costs, and the dental hygienist may be able to work two or three days in the same office. This can be advantageous, as the opportunity to acquire an immediate position may be easier and new graduates are providing preventive oral health care to an area that may have difficulty getting dental hygienists to commute or relocate. These factors may be negotiating points with the employer, and is discussed later in this chapter.

WORKING AS A TEMPORARY

Temporary employment is another avenue for an immediate position if the dental hygienist resides in an area where job openings occur less frequently. Furthermore, this can be an excellent avenue for steady yet flexible employment. Many practices are opting to schedule advance appointments for dental hygiene patients. This means the dental hygienist can be scheduled three to six months in advance. Unless vacations are pre-blocked in the schedule, the dental hygienist may find it difficult to take time off from work. In addition, when time off is taken in the hygiene department, the practice may see a decrease in production and collections, since fewer patients are scheduled.

One way to alleviate down time for the practice is to hire a *temporary* during regular staff vacations or extended periods of absence, such as maternity leaves. By doing this, the practice makes a positive business decision, as it will not have to reschedule patients. Temporary employees have the opportunity to work in many environments for short periods of time.

Many communities have agencies that specialize in dental personnel, offering the new graduate the opportunity to market himself or herself as a temporary employee. Working with a temporary agency is another way to gain employment, and for many, working as a "temp" is a viable source of regular employment and income. The value of marketing and public relations skills is certainly applicable to this type of situation. Compensation may be handled differently under temporary positions; thus, consult a tax accountant on what is expected for temporary employment.

There are many advantages to beginning a new career in a temporary position. The new practitioner is able to test numerous dental practices. When unsure as to what type of office environment you seek, temporary positions will allow you to work with many offices, their staff members, and their patients. This way, if the environment in not compatible with the way you had planned on practicing your discipline, it becomes easy to move onto the next position.

The disadvantage is that there may be times when the clinician is unsure as to when the next position will present itself. However, this may be a small inconvenience when evaluating the advantages.

EMPLOYMENT RESOURCES

New graduates may be unfamiliar with where or how to seek employment. Many dental practices will submit flyers to dental hygiene programs and request placement on the career bulletin board. This is one resource to investigate before leaving school. As mentioned, seeking career information through ADHA is the first step to finding the position that suits each dental hygienist. Other resources include state and local dental hygiene organizations, local dental organizations, practicing professionals, dental assistants, the classified ads, professional journal advertisements, and employment agencies. The Internet is fast becoming a valuable resource for numerous needs in the career industry (keyword: *job search*). Resources are plentiful and assist in getting started in a career search.

PREPARING FOR INTERVIEWS

After taking clinical board examinations and prior to receiving a license to practice, dental hygiene graduates may be interviewing with potential employers in areas they think they may want to practice. During interviews with possible employers, many new graduates are so overwhelmed at beginning their new career, they often miss information being presented and miss the opportunity to ask important questions that may help them understand what a new employer expects.

When entering a practice for a scheduled interview, the applicant immediately notices the environment, the office décor, atmosphere, and how modern the equipment may be. Often, a new dental hygienist visualizes himself or herself in the new working environment and wants to be sure he or she will be comfortable in that particular environment. Providing dental hygiene services, education, and motivation to patients in each practice is the basis of the education and training. However, during that interview process, numerous subjects may not be discussed due to time constraints (the dentist may be interviewing during working hours and between patients) or neither party is fully prepared to discuss important information related to the open position. Most importantly, employers have expectations that new dental hygienists may not be aware. Many of these expectations underlie the association of employees with the practice and often go unrealized.

When initiating a career search, endless hours will be spent if the search is to be successful. Each interview becomes critical in moving forward to the goal of that first position. For those who interview frequently, job offers should be expected. If the resumes and letters of interest are not getting you an interview, then reevaluation of the search strategy becomes necessary. Preparation is essential to eliminating stress.

Interviewing skills are key factors in selecting the person who will fit into a practice. The main purpose for interviewing is for the dental hygienist and the potential employer to learn about each other. Formats range from telephone interviews to panel interviews to personal settings. No matter the form, the process remains similar.

It is important to be prepared with your own expectations and questions when interviewing with potential employers. What is the best approach to interviews when seeking the first or tenth career position? Taking the interview process in steps will help the applicant anticipate questions that may be asked by employers and prepare questions to ask of prospective employers.

Using some principles of Stephen R. Covey's habits from *The 7 Habits of Highly Effective People,* we can see how certain aspects may be applied to dental hygiene interview techniques.

1. **Be Proactive.**

   Essentially, this means to take initiative and responsibility for yourself. Generally, most people are reactive to their surroundings and the things that happen to them. With increased knowledge in business and management, being proactive allows you to stand out and be seen as a leader.

   Being proactive in an interview situation, the new employee would initiate pertinent questions applicable to duties that may be performed if employed with the office. For example, dentists generally ask how a dental hygienist determines the need for root planing procedures. When taking a proactive approach to interview questions, the employee might be the one to ask how the office determines root planing procedures and what the policy is for referrals to a specialist.

2. **Begin with the end in mind.**

   Where do you want to be next year at this time? What type of practice do you want to be associated with? Some things to consider when interviewing include
   - Informal/formal environment
   - Casual personalities
   - Open communication
   - Oral health care philosophy

   Knowing what type of environment you want to be working in at a future date will help you decide what type of practice you want to work with.

3. **The win-win outcome.**

   Many new graduates may not be hired after an interview and feel as though they lost to someone who may have had better qualifications. When interviewees are not hired, there is always something gained from the interview, as it is a learning experience. Covey (1990) explains that the win-win situation is a frame of heart and mind seeking the benefit of all interactions (p. 207). So, no matter the outcome, there is a learned experience that becomes incorporated into each person's background that may be of benefit at a later point in time.

Interviewing can be an arduous task for the practice and a nerve-racking experience for a new dental hygiene graduate. By taking the time to incorporate appropriate information and develop new tools that can be of use, all experiences have a positive outcome.

The Employer's Interview

Selecting the right person for employment is a skill that may take years to develop. Employers become frustrated when the turnover rate in their practice is high and they go through employees every six months. Changes in any practice can be expensive, annoying, and frustrating to each staff member. For new dental hygiene graduates, having an understanding of what the employer must consider will be of benefit when preparing for interviews. Some considerations by the employer may include

- Determining the level of competency needed for the open position
- Preparing a job description to orient the new employee
- Explaining the job requirements during the interview
- Accurately observing the person being interviewed
- Evaluating the responses from the prospective employee

In addition, the employer and potential employee must be aware of the legal aspects of the interview process. Every state has laws against discrimination. These laws must also be adhered to during interviews. Questions in an interview process cannot include

- Those related to race or color
- Those related to gender or religion
- Those related to marital status or age
- Those related to military status
- Those related to national origin or residency (In 1986 the Immigration Reform and Control Act specified requirements for new em-

ployees to complete an I-9 form. This form was designed to prevent the employment of illegal aliens.)

Social security numbers are also matters of personal information. Many organizations have begun to eliminate the use of social security numbers as a form of identification, opting for use of randomly selected numbers.

Now that some groundwork has been explained and defined, what types of questions could an employer ask, and what might the employer be looking for in a new employee? How might the actual interview take place?

Most employers will do their best to keep the interview relaxed and comfortable. This helps to bring out true personalities and may encourage more self-disclosure from both parties. Easy questions regarding personal and professional behavior are typically used to initiate the session

- How would you describe yourself in a working environment?
- Why do you feel you would like to work with this practice?
- Why did you leave your last position?
- Can you handle constructive criticism?
- How would you handle questions about fees from your patients?
- How would you handle an irate patient?
- What salary range are you expecting?
- What specialized qualifications or education do you possess?

Employers expect a positive attitude in any prospective employee. Promptness is observed the first time you enter the practice. Do not arrive late for any interview.

Of course, each employer and each interview will be unique to their respective practices. Some interviews will include the business or office manager. Furthermore, some interviews are handled exclusively by the office or business manager. This is similar to a screening technique. If the office manager conducts interviews, the employer may only re-interview when the potential candidates have been selected.

During each interview, be sure to listen carefully to the questions being asked. Answers should focus on your qualifications, special skills, and education. You may focus on aspects dental hygiene courses that you feel contributed to your strong points or that held a particular interest for you. Make sure to emphasize the potential benefits you feel you can bring to the practice. Interjecting personal information is fine, but be sure not to dwell too long on the topic.

Your Interview

While in dental hygiene school, many students envision what they would like as they begin their career. What will the appointments be like? Will new graduates be given a full hour for each appointment, or does the practice expect the entering dental hygienist to manage within the same timeframe as the person who has been with the practice for several years? Does everyone expect to begin his or her new career in the ideal working environment?

As interviews begin, new licentiates will want to develop an outline of their own expectations or perhaps of the environment in which they prefer to work. Salary is likely the most common topic on the minds of both the employer and the applicant. Yet if questions arise on what you expect as a starting wage, you will want to have a figure ready to present to the dentist or potential employer. Research this figure through various avenues. Contact the state local dental hygiene association for the most recent information on salary ranges in your area. There will be many topics such as this that you will want to research. Be prepared with pertinent questions for the employer so that accepting a position is based on complete information about the practice and the duties expected of you.

How about questions to ask the employer? In order to present yourself professionally, there are also questions you should avoid. For example, do not

- ask what they can offer you.
- ask what the top pay rate is in the office.
- ask if your schedule can be altered for your child's afterschool activities.
- state that you have no questions at all.

Skill and technique are important when beginning to interview. Many interviews contribute to improving skills.

Another aspect to avoid is appearing desperate for a position. When new practitioners present themselves in this manner, they are likely to engage certain pitfalls of employment. Pitfalls include a lower than average wage, fewer benefits if applicable, fewer workdays, or perhaps longer working hours. These things can happen to anyone when unprepared.

Examples of questions to ask the interviewer include

A. **Clinical concerns**
   1. What kinds of instruments are used in the office?
   2. Is the employer willing to order instruments?

3. Are instruments shared among the dental hygienists in the office?
4. Who makes the dental hygiene diagnosis and treatment plan?
5. What is the protocol for referrals to specialists?
6. What sterilization methods are employed?
7. To what extent are OSHA standards practiced?

B. **Scheduling**
1. Who schedules dental hygiene appointments?
2. What recall system is practiced?
3. What is expected when patients fail appointments?
4. How long are hygiene appointments? (45 or 60 minutes)

C. **General practice information**
1. What constitutes full time and part time?
2. What is the negotiable salary range?
3. Does the office pay for continuing education courses?
4. How is the computer system applied to hygiene services?
5. What benefits are available to the dental hygienist?
6. Does the staff work when the dentist is out of the office?
7. How interactive are staff meetings, and how often are they held?
8. What is the channel of communication or command?

These are only some of the questions new graduates can incorporate into an interview. Keep in mind that presenting yourself as an experienced professional will be advantageous to potential employers. Thus planning for questions is essential to the overall presentation. Communicating with dental hygienists who work or have worked in the office is recommended, as they can offer another perspective on the operations and working personalities of the practice. In the employment interview, questions from new graduates are valid and will assist them in making the decision to become employed in that particular office.

The Working Interview

Employers will often want to try the dental hygienist before actually hiring him or her on a permanent basis. Working interviews may consist of one full or half day or even a few weeks of providing clinical services to the patients. The dental hygienist is compensated for these services and will want to fully understand when the pay period occurs and how much the pay will be for the time period agreed upon. Advantages of a working interview for the employer include being able to indirectly observe clinical skills, interpersonal skills with patients, and relationship skills with coworkers. The advantages for the dental hygienist include being able to observe how the staff interacts with them and others, how staff interacts with patients, and how everyone interacts with the employer. Another advantage for the dental hygienist is that he or she is able to work with the equipment and instruments that are currently in the practice. This will provide information on what may need replacement or must be purchased should they decide to take this position. He or she can also determine whether or not the time allotment for each patient is sufficient and whether there is pressure to stay on time. How receptive is the staff to questions when the new employee is uncertain of office procedures or locating materials?

Working interviews may be more of an advantage than many may think. Most new employees are excited about being hired for a permanent position, only to realize a few weeks later that working philosophies or do not mesh or other negative issues exist. New practitioners have nothing to lose, as compensation is given for their time. When unsure as to whether to accept a position, suggest a working interview to the employer.

Interviews and Personality Tests

Although rare, there are employers who have applicants take a personality test. Not all personality tests are written. Some are verbal; thus you may be unaware this test is being given. Personality tests are designed to assist in identifying certain behaviors, habits, or patterns held by a person. Verbal interviews can consist of specific questions that have been designed to promote certain responses from the applicant. Thus the employer is able to determine your capacity to fit into his or her practice based on your responses. If the employer has used the same technique on every employee hired, the personality of the practice becomes homogenous in nature, which may make a smooth working environment. As with other aspects associated with job searching, personality tests will also have advantages and disadvantages. When thoroughly prepared for interviews, the professional personality will be expressed naturally.

Attire

Now that some time has been spent getting all the professional information ready to present to potential employers, what clothing is most appropriate for interviews? There are no absolutes for proper dress. However, keep in mind the environment in which the interview will take place. If you are meeting the employer during office hours, you may choose to wear something more professional. This does not mean clinic attire is required. Most often, a business-like approach is best. A business suit makes a professional statement. More and more, dentists may be dropping the white shirt and tie for casual polo shirts or scrubs. However, as a potential new employee, a professional approach makes a better impression. Avoid wearing an outfit if you question its appropriateness: sundresses, sandals, and so on. Men may opt for shirts and ties.

Grooming is another factor where image will be represented. If you feel good, you will look good. Pay attention to hairstyles and makeup (for women). Keep it professional, as in your dental hygiene education. Overall appearance is what the employer and staff observe first. Make a good first impression, while feeling confident and comfortable. Neat and clean is the best approach.

Resumes

Now that you have prepared yourself for the interviews, the next important step is to be sure that the resume is in order. Writing a **resume** can be a difficult task, but for many it is the opportunity to identify and promote their talents and skills. Presenting a resume is presenting a brief statement of employment experience and education. As learned, public relations entails dealing with image. Dental hygiene graduates are able to apply the idea of image in promoting the highest aspects of their qualifications.

Many resume formats are easily found and standard in computer software. Some programs include resumes in the word or publishing programs. They are preformatted so all that is required is filling in the blanks. A variety of formats, including traditional, professional, and contemporary, allow each person to express individuality. Once created, the resume can be printed on a high-quality bond paper. Additional resources for resumes are resume services and local printing or copying businesses, as well as the Internet (key word: *resume*). Some firms may have computers available for customers to format their own document.

Resumes are a brief summary of qualifications and skills. Usually, this is accomplished in one page. Should a resume extend longer than one page, there is the possibility that only the first page gets read or the employer skims for pertinent information. Be concise with qualifications, but be sure to highlight special aspects that may stand above others applying for the same position. Resumes should be typed, using a computer or typewriter, or typeset by a professional printer. The font chosen for resumes need to be easily read. Avoid being too elaborate, as this can distract from the information presented. Always proofread and reread the final product. Avoid grammatical errors and spelling errors. Computer programs are extremely useful, but they are not perfect. It is often helpful to have another person proofread the resume and point out errors or make suggestions when information lacks clarity.

How can your resume stand out among the others?

1. **Focus on the content.** If an employer does not have time to read resumes, there is a chance they may quickly glance through the form and decide on who to interview within a matter of seconds. Past experience can play a major part in such a decision. Highlight your best abilities and accomplishments.
2. **Visual Appearance.** If the resume is to get more than a few seconds of attention, it should catch the eye. Color, bullets, borders, spacing, italicizing, and style will add to the presentation of the resume. Make sure the printer cartridge is new and the printed resume is clean.
3. **Be accurate, concise, and clear.** List items and accomplishments first so that the reader's attention stays focused. No one wants to search for information that is buried in the "fluff." Interest will be lost quickly, and your resume may find the shredder.
4. **Use an appropriate font and high quality paper.** White, cream, and light blues or grays have shown to be most appealing to readers—nothing fancy, just quality. As mentioned, the font size should be easily read. Type size 12 is widely accepted, and 14 may be too large, as it appears you may want to lengthen the document. Type size 10 may be used for sections, but many times it is too small for easy reading.
5. **Proofread and edit.** This may be the most difficult task to accomplish. Mistakes are often overlooked because the information is so familiar to the writer. Have someone else proofread for errors and comprehension. Do not send a resume with typos, spelling errors, or whiteout corrections. The goal is perfection and professionalism.

Resumes may include the following sections:

• **Objective Statement.** This is a brief statement that targets reasons for seeking employment in a particular practice or setting. Usually, it is goal-oriented. State the goals you seek on a professional and personal level by being associated with the dentist or practice.

- **Experience.** Depending on the amount and scope of experience, include previous jobs that augment the skills required for the new position. Begin with the most recent. Include each employer's name and address and a short description of duties performed in the position.
- **Education.** Depending on the age of the graduate, the farthest one may want to go back is high school. More importantly, list all college education, degrees, honors, and awards received. Some may choose to include GPA information; however, many find it is not necessary. For those who attend special workshops or continuing education seminars that are relevant to the career, is it a good idea to include this information.
- **Professional memberships.** If previously licensed or a member of a professional organization, include this in the resume. This indicates activity and interest in the profession and issues that may affect your career or community.
- **Credentials/licensure.** Include all information about your licensure and credentials. If you possess a dental assisting license, list it. Provide the year in which it was received and the license number itself. If you hold other certificates, such as CPR, be sure to include them. Furthermore, extract any expanded functions affiliated with a dental hygiene license, such as nitrous oxide sedation and local anesthesia. Many states may not include this with the dental hygiene licensure, but if your state does, be sure to highlight those skills.
- **Personal data.** It is often advantageous to include information on hobbies, community activities, and family interests. This may give some insight about how you may prioritize aspects of your lifestyle.
- **References.** References are generally provided upon request. These will include coworkers or personal friends who can attest to your character and to the benefits of having you as an employee. Be sure to select those you prefer to have the potential employer contact, as many employers take the time to call those you have listed.

Resume styles will differ; however, they will hold the same essential information. The sample resume in Figure 10–1 represents some of the information that can be incorporated to provide the appropriate information for the position you are seeking to fill.

Depending on your past experience and the extent of your education, the resume will vary in length. Be sure to include all pertinent information, including professional memberships and volunteer programs.

55 Hilltop Avenue Riverview   555-0101 / sanderson @internet.net

Suzanne Anderson, RDH

Objective	To obtain employment in a progressive environment that promotes quality oral health and provides open communication for new ideas.
Experience	1998–1999 James Jones, DDS, General Dentistry Southridge, SC **Chairside Assitant** • Four-handed dentistry • OSHA monitor • Clinical inventory
	1997–1999 Ferguson, DDS and Bardell DDS Southridge, SC **Insurance Coordinator** • Daily insurance processing / claims
Education	1998–2000 Southridge Community College, SC • A.S. Dental Hygiene - Honors • 1992 B.S. Biology, Southridge State College, SC
	LICENSURE: 2000 DH State License # 55551. Skilled in clinical aspects of debridement, root planing, local anesthesia, nitrous oxide sedation, sealant placement, periodontal assessment, treatment planning, and patient education.
Professional Memberships	• Member- American Dental Hygienists' Association • SCC Alumni Association
Community Work	• Volunteer for county school screenings • Oral health fair • Tobacco cessation presentation
Interests	Outdoor activities, horseback riding, water sports.
REFERENCES	Available upon request.

Figure 10–1 A sample resume.

THE COVER LETTER

A *cover letter* (see Figure 10–2) should accompany your resume. There are several types of cover letters that can be employed. If the practice has asked for a resume, the cover letter will want to address the request. If sending resumes as a "cold contact," the focus is on identifying the qualifications needed for the dental hygiene position. Additionally, if someone has referred you to a specific office, the cover letter should mention the individual who made the referral. It is a good idea to individualize each cover letter to the dentist or practice you are applying to. Cover letters allow you to introduce yourself. The letter may include identifying the practice's need for a certain quality or skill, while pointing out that you may be the one to meet that need.

July 16, 2000

Suzanne Anderson, RDH
55 Hilltop Avenue
Riverview, California
(101) 555-0101
email: sanderson@internet.net

Dear Dr. Wells,

    Enclosed please find my resume submitted in response to the position you are seeking to fill. My current goals include participating in patient education and promotion of optimal oral health, while working in an atmosphere that provides a free exchange of ideas.
    Upon review of my resume, I am confident you will find I possess the skills necessary to enhance your dental team. In addition, I hope to provide organizational skills and extensive patient education to your practice.
    I look forward to meeting you and your staff at your earliest convenience. You may contact me at the address listed above.
    Thank you for your consideration.

Sincerely,
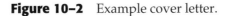
Suzanne Anderson, RDH
Suzanne Anderson, RDH

Figure 10–2 Example cover letter.

Avoid replicating information that is found in the resume itself. Cover letters are brief and may consist of one to three paragraphs. The first paragraph should state the reason for submitting the resume for the position. You may also want to mention how you learned of the position. The second paragraph should explain the reason(s) for your interest in working with this practice and point out why you are the person for the position. The third paragraph can suggest meeting the employer in person and provide information on your availability or flexibility regarding the employer's schedule. Be sure to mention that there will be a follow-up on this communication. Finally, thank the employer for the opportunity and for his or her time in reviewing the resume.

Post-Interview Acknowledgments

After interviewing with potential employers, sending a note of gratitude (see Figure 10–3) is considered courteous and is appreciated by employers and staff members who may have been involved in the interview process. This is also seen as a good marketing tool. The dental hygienist has acknowledged the time spent by the employer and reminded him or her of the meeting. It is also a great opportunity to market your skills and refresh the employer's memory on the interview. Thank-you letters can

---

Dear Dr. Wells,

I appreciated having the opportunity to meet with you and your staff. I also appreciate the information you provided regarding your philosophy for dental care.

I am greatly interested in working with you and your patients, and feel I meet the qualifications you seek in a dental hygienist.

I will contact your office next Tuesday to learn of your decision.

Sincerely,
Suzanne Anderson, RDH
Suzanne Anderson, RDH

Figure 10–3 Example of a thank-you letter.

be formal or simple. Specific points to consider for thank-you letters include

1. Be brief.
2. Restate your interest in the position.
3. It can be used as the follow-up contact.
4. Restate your qualifications.

BEGINNING THE NEW JOB

Once the interviews have ended and the job offer is accepted, there are new aspects of employment and working in the dental hygiene profession that new practitioners will want to be informed. Policy manuals, probationary periods, compensation types, and more are items not usually discussed during interviews. Additionally, many seasoned dental hygienists have indicated that negotiating skills would have helped them many times when it came to benefits. Once the decision has been made to accept a position, the new dental hygienist will want to be prepared for the next phase of beginning the new job.

Most new positions come with the understanding that a probationary period exists. This means that for a designated time (30 to 90 days), the new employee can leave the job at any time without stating a specific reason. During the probationary period, the employer also has the opportunity to terminate the agreement at any time. Most often, this time period allows the employer to withhold benefits (if applicable) until both parties agree that the employment relationship will be extended, indefinitely.

Compensation

Compensation is something that most new graduates look forward to as a dental hygienist. It is no secret that the compensation rate is attractive. However, there are many ways to be compensated as a dental hygienist. Salaries will range all over the country and within the state where you reside. Currently, salary ranges can be found by contacting your local or state dental hygiene association. Some of the ways the practitioner can be compensated are found in Table 10–1.

There are likely other ways to be compensated as a dental hygienist; however, these examples will give the new employee something to consider, based upon the type of practice. However you choose to be com-

Table 10–1   Examples of Compensation for the Dental Hygienist

Type of Compensation	Description
Daily	The dental hygienist is paid a flat rate regardless of how much production is gained or the number of patients seen that day.
Base pay with commission	This means the practitioner will receive a base amount no matter what happens with scheduling. Any amount produced by the clinician over the base rate will be the amount of compensation for that day. For example, the base rate might be $200. Depending on the type of procedures scheduled, the production may have amounted to $950 for the day. If the commission is 40% of anything over the $200, the compensation for that day amounts to $300. This is the amount paid to the dental hygienist. Thus, the daily pay rate will vary.
Hourly	Hourly is based on a flat rate for the number of hours worked.
Commission only	This means that the dental hygienist has agreed to work for a certain commission. Thus, no matter how many patients are seen or the type of treatment given, the daily rate is based on total production each day.
Commission on procedures	This is based on certain procedures being compensated over the agreed salary, whether it's a daily rate or not. For example, if the clinician performs four root-planing cases in a day, the compensation is extra based upon the agreement with the employer. Perhaps the dental hygienist receives an extra $30 per case. If the daily rate for compensation was $250, another $120 would be received for that day.

pensated, be very clear on the terms of the agreement. The bottom line is to be paid what you are worth. Many articles about compensation can be found in dental hygiene publications, professional organizations offer plentiful resources.

Another aspect of compensation is an annual salary increase. More often than not, the dental hygienist is not included in annual increases, due to the amount he or she is already paid. However, is this fair to any employee? This is an issue you may not be comfortable addressing at the start of a new job, but it is important to find out how the practice handles salary increases for its staff members. By addressing the question early, the professional dental hygienist can learn how to approach the subject in a timely manner. Most employers will not bring the subject up on a regular basis, so the employee must act in his or her own interest. According to a 1998 forecast by the Department of Labor, the number of dental hygienists is expected to increase 41 percent through the year 2005. The number of new programs opening on an annual basis indicates this growth. Many practices offer **merit** raises, which are based on the employee's performance and skills. Merit raises can occur annually or at the discretion of the employer. **Cost-of-living** raises may not be provided in many practices. These increases would also occur annually. They are based on the average cost it takes to maintain a standard of living (for example food, clothing, and medical expenses). Salary increases is a topic that any new employee will want to fully understand. Any time a salary increase is indicated and requested, be prepared to justify the increase.

Justification may include increased production in the dental hygiene department, broader responsibilities in the department, or for the simple fact that you have been employed in the same office for several years. If increases are not provided for the dental hygienist, it can be something to negotiate at different points in your association with any practice.

Benefits

Benefits are likely the most important area for the dental hygienist to consider when seeking a position. As you may already know from many conversations with licensed practitioners and your instructors, **benefits** can be difficult to find for the dental hygienist. This is one area where many have voiced the need for negotiating tips so that some benefits are realized during their career. Although there are dental hygiene positions that provide full benefits, such as those in education, public health, corporate environments, and some private practice positions, these benefits are provided for full-time employment. Full time is generally defined as at least 32 hours per week. As mentioned, most dental hygienists prefer to work part time. A good benefit package may cost the employer approximately 20 percent of the employee's salary. Depending on the size of the practice, benefits can be expensive to the practice. Keep in mind that most dental practices are small businesses. Although benefits can vary widely, the major components will include

- Medical and dental
- Sick days and well days
- Holidays
- Continuing education
- Bonus incentives
- Profit sharing
- Retirement plans

How would this break down from an employer's perspective? Using an example from *RDH* magazine, a benefit package based on an annual salary of $30,000 may look like that presented in Table 10–2.

Since benefits vary region to region and on an individual basis, this represents only a sample of what the employer must spend to provide a package to employees. Dental hygienists can use this information to their advantage, as many will be able to negotiate portions of a benefit package and enhance their compensation.

Another example for discussing benefits up front is holidays. For many dental hygienists, the holidays can require advanced planning. Many practices choose to take several days off during the holidays. Legal holidays typically fall on Monday throughout the year. Be sure to ask what is the normal practice for the office during these times. If unable to take the same amount of time off, working as a substitute or temporary

Table 10–2 Sample Benefit Package

Benefit	Cost to Employer
2-week vacation/year	$ 1,200
5 sick days	$ 600
Health insurance	$ 136/month
Continuing education	$ 400
Uniform allowance	$ 50/month
Free dental care	$ 220
Bonus - production	$ 219/month
TOTAL package	**$ 7,280/year**

Source: RDH Magazine, June 1998

can alleviate loss of income during holidays. Other benefits such as medical and dental are more difficult, but are available depending on the type of dental hygiene environment one chooses to be employed.

Negotiating

What will it take to incorporate negotiating skills? Negotiating is not in the comfort zone for many individuals. Since the majority of dental hygienists are women, it becomes an aspect that even fewer are comfortable in implementing. Negotiating often has more to do with being a newcomer and having no leverage than with being a woman. Julie Nierenberg, coauthor of *Women and the Art of Negotiation,* states that "One of the most overlooked features of negotiating successfully is trying to figure everything from the other point of view. We're so stuck in our own point of view that we don't stop to consider, how will they look at all of this?" Therefore, to gain any aspect of benefits, the big picture is what each new employee must keep in mind. Numerous books and Internet resources are available to those who seek more information about negotiating skills (keyword: *negotiating skills*). However, some of the basics can be provided in order for students and new graduates to familiarize themselves with the process.

A. **Your negotiation.**
   - No two experiences are alike due to the differences in your needs, the market, and where you are in your career.
B. **Do your research.**
   - Will the employer negotiate?
   - Who is the decision maker?
C. **Know your priorities.**
   - Is it salary, benefits, bonuses?
D. **Stay focused on long-term goals.**
   - Will tradeoffs occur?
   - Be ready to justify your needs and requirements.
   - Compare your career or job to others that include benefits.

Source: Kimberly Wandel, *Wisdom Technologies*

Approach is another aspect of negotiating that requires attention. During the interview, keep in mind that the office wants to hire you. As health care providers, both parties share the same goal. Flexibility must be exercised, and each person must remain honest and fair. If benefit requests are not met on the first attempt, inquire as to when they can be revisited. If the practice is observant of annual employee evaluations, the next benefit on the list can be discussed at that time. The most important aspect to remember is that you must be willing to walk away. Even as a new graduate and a new employee, there are many positions available. To be successful at negotiating benefits, whether it is one benefit or an entire package, walking away is something to be prepared for.

When negotiating benefits, keep in mind even seemingly minor items. For example, if you accept a position out of your immediate community and commuting is required, how about negotiating for gas expense? It may not take into account the wear and tear on your vehicle, but it will assist in the costs for fuel. Over time, this expense adds up. This is the first step in negotiating benefits. As experience is gained, the dental hygienist becomes more in tune to what he or she seeks in a benefits package. If benefits are never an option for the dental hygienist, taking small steps is the next best option.

EMPLOYMENT CONTRACTS

Some practices extend an employment contract to their employees. This type of contract can be advantageous to both the employer and the employee, as it helps to eliminate possible misunderstandings of expectations on both sides. Employment contracts will have numerous categories, and you should carefully review the contract if presented by the employer. These contracts are another area for negotiation. They can also be presented by the dental hygienist, as they are not limited to employers in their creation. Most employment contracts will cover topics such as

- Position and duties to be performed
- Work schedule
- Compensation: amount and how the compensation is paid
- Pay schedule
- Benefits and how they are deducted from a paycheck
- Evaluation periods
- Salary increase schedule/type of increase (e.g., cost of living/merit)
- Fringe benefits (e.g., continuing education uniform)
- Vacations/holidays
- Termination of employment methods/process

POLICY MANUALS

Office **policy manuals** are likely to be found in most practices. It is of benefit for the office to have them on hand and to provide a copy for all staff members. They assist is decreasing misunderstandings about what the practice will provide to its staff members as well as expectations it has of employees. Policy manuals will range in complexity, again based on the size and scope of the practice. However, basic ingredients will be found in all manuals.

A. **Terms of employment:** This section describes the type of employment offered
   - Equal opportunity
   - At-will (termination can come from either party at any time for any reason)
   - Sexual harassment policy

B. **General Employment Definitions/Requirements**
   - Full time/part time (defined)
   - Temporary (defined)
   - Waiting period determined prior to onset of benefits
   - License requirements/maintaining licensure

C. **Work Schedule**
   - Office hours
   - Individual work schedules
   - When doctors are out of the office
   - Time cards/tardiness
   - Lunch breaks/breaks
   - Staff meetings

D. **Compensation Issues**
   - Types of compensation
   - Flexible work arrangements
   - Overtime duties/compensation
   - Bonus pay/severance pay
   - Pay periods/salary advances
   - Performance evaluations
   - Job abandonment (termination without notice)

E. **Employee Benefits**
   - Vacations/holidays
   - Sick time
   - Health insurance/dental benefits

- Continuing education
- Worker's compensation
- Jury duty
- Leaves of absence
- Bereavement leave
- Pregnancy leave

F. **Dress and Appearance**
  - Personal hygiene
  - Hair
  - Nails
  - Jewelry
  - Gum chewing
  - Shoes
  - Uniform attire

G. **Additional sections**
  - Conduct during work
  - Personal business on company time
  - Office supplies
  - Confidentiality
  - Noncompetition clauses (competing for business from patients while at work) Example: Many offices have lunch rooms or break rooms where staff and patients may leave merchandise catalogs, and staff is able to purchase goods via mail order.

Many categories in employment contracts and office policy manuals are similar. They are all designed to inform staff members of expectations and to decrease misunderstandings during employment with the practice. Employment contracts for the dental hygienist or any employee are helpful in that they bind the employer to follow through with all items that have been agreed upon.

Evaluations are provided for the staff members, typically on an annual basis, so that employees can be informed of their strong points, areas where improvement might be necessary, and for both the employer and employee to discuss other aspects of the duties. Dental hygienists may not participate in an evaluation, but many feel this would benefit the professional working relationship. One reason the dental hygienists may not be provided evaluations is because regular salary increases may not be included during employment. However, it gives both the dentist and the dental hygienist a chance to discuss philosophy, new programs that have entered the practice for the patient, and essentially to touch base on operations. During the interview process or shortly after beginning a new position, inquire as to the evaluation process in the office and ask to participate. It is an advantage for the professional to continuously provide information as well as participate in changes that occur in the office. Evaluations are one avenue that can be utilized by the dental hygienist.

SUMMARY

Job searching requires thoughtful planning. The availability of dental hygiene positions must be considered when initiating the search. Some find they begin by commuting to outlying areas, and some find they prefer to relocate to new communities. Working as a temporary can be a source of stable income as well as a flexible choice for employment.

Interviews are done by employers and should also be conducted by the potential employee. Three key characteristics can be incorporated to assist in active participation of interviews: being proactive, looking at the end result, and the desire of a win-win outcome. Gaining employment may also consist of personality tests, employment testing, and numerous questions on professional and personal aspects. Working interviews can be advantageous for both the applicant and the employer, as it allows each person to work with the other to determine if their philosophies mesh.

Resumes are necessary to promote skills and qualifications. Formats are easily available and numerous other avenues are readily available to insure a quality document. Resumes will contain specific sections with concise information for any potential employer to review easily. Typically, cover letters accompany all resumes, and sending a post-interview acknowledgment is another way to remind the employer of the meeting.

Compensation comes in many forms. The new graduate will want to carefully review what is being offered and how it will fit into his or her plan as a professional. Everything is negotiable, and incorporating some skills will assist in obtaining the overall goal as the career begins. Benefits are also negotiable, and there are some dental hygiene positions that provide full benefits. Clinicians are encouraged to expand and seek positions that enhance the clinical aspect of their career.

Policy manuals are found in nearly all practices and are provided to inform staff members of the benefits provided as well as to define each person's duties. It will also define the parameters for leaves of absence and worker's compensation.

1. In this group exercise, one group member is seeking employment in one of the environments listed below. Create a list of questions that will be used during an interview with the potential employer. Be sure to design questions that target the practice environment chosen. In addition, a second group member can prepare questions as if he or she were the employer. At the end of the exercise, role-play an interview session.
   A. General practice
   B. Periodontal practice
   C. Pedodontic practice
   D. Community dental clinic
   E. Federal Indian reservation
   F. Hospital dental provider (providing dental hygiene services to developmentally disabled)

2. Create a resume that you will use when you begin seeking employment. Be sure to include all sections pertinent to your experience and education, as well as references. Be sure to create a cover letter and a post-interview acknowledgment.

3. As a dental hygienist in a new practice, you have been asked to create a section of the policy manual that will address all dental hygienists employed by the practice. Provide the information required for the policy manual. Be sure to address working hours and days, compensation methods, and benefits that will apply.

4. Identify and briefly explain the types of salary increases that may occur in the dental practice.

11

Planning for the Future and Career Longevity

OBJECTIVES

Upon reading the material in this chapter, you will be able to

1. Describe the differences between stocks, mutual funds, and IRAs.
2. Explain the meaning of portfolio.
3. Describe CD investments.
4. Explain liability insurance.
5. Explain disability insurance.
6. Identify the need for self-care and physical health.
7. Describe the benefits of professional membership.

INTRODUCTION

As students graduate and enter a field of flexibility and financial independence, getting a head start on retirement through wise investment strategies is the next step in continuing education. At the end of 1999, social security funds and the assurance that there would be enough funds to support the vast "babyboomer" population was in great question. No one is sure that the monies deducted from your paycheck each month will be available for your financial support upon retiring. If you are still 10 to 15 years from retirement, social security funds may be depleted by the time you are eligible to collect. Annual statements are sent by the Social Security Administration, documenting the funds you have contributed and what your monthly benefit is expected to be upon retirement. Due to the instability of social security, it is wise for the new graduate (regardless of age) to begin an investment **portfolio** (a summary of all investments held) so that retirement includes some financial security. Not only is retirement a good reason to invest, but many dental hygienists will want to send their children to college, purchase a vacation home, or just be assured of financial security. Essentially, you want to invest in something that will assist in creating wealth.

Financial planners look at the earning periods of an individual's career and lifetime. According to many planners, there are three periods to consider: age 24 to 45, when people accumulate not only money but material items; age 45 to 65, when most working persons are well established in their careers; and age 65 and up, when the majority of working persons are retired or semiretired. Regardless of your age when beginning a dental hygiene career, consideration must be given to the amount of money required when retirement does come. It is wise to save funds on a regular basis and to seek investments that will generate the most interest for hard-earned dollars. Furthermore, inflation and the cost of living must be taken into account from start to retirement. Consideration must also be given to life expectancy after retirement.

When considering investments or savings accounts, be sure to spend some time investigating the returns given on the initial investment. For example, most banking institutions only pay 3 to 5 percent interest per year on a regular savings account. Therefore, if $2,000 is placed in the account and nothing is added for the year, the return would range from $60 to $100. Not much, for hard-earned dollars. However, if that same $2,000 was placed into the stock market in conservative areas where 11 percent could be earned, the return could be $220, and after 30 years, the investment is worth $53,416.19 (The Motley Fool, 1999). Given this information, it is wise to find an investment broker that will assist in the type of funds that will achieve the goals desired, no matter what you save for.

THE BASICS OF INVESTING

Financial planning means looking at your personal situation, outlining your goals, and developing an action plan that will achieve those goals. By doing so, you can remain focused on the success of the outcome. When initiating an investment plan, financial firm Morgan Stanley advises, take time to outline some basic steps:

- Identify, prioritize, and quantify financial goals and objectives. Begin by listing goals you want to accomplish: an individual retirement plan, a college fund, etc.
- Summarize personal data and records so that they are easy to follow. Develop a file that includes the type of investments owned, and frequently update it to display **net worth** (amount of money remaining after all debts are paid).
- Compare goals to investments. Be sure that your investments are working to their best ability, the interest rate still competitive, and the investment still viable.
- Develop a savings and investment plan that is specific to your needs. It may include mutual funds, stocks, and certificates of deposit.
- Monitor progress on a regular basis.

There are numerous avenues available for investors. Thus, it is easy to get started while becoming more familiar with the different markets. Table 11–1 summarizes some of these avenues.

Compounding interest is meant to be an advantage if you are attentive to how it works. Compounding interest adds to the initial investment due to the rate of the interest and the amount of time that the funds remain untouched. The more you can put away into a savings account and not touch until retirement, the faster the funds grow because of the interest gained year after year. Thus, the power of compounding will be the most important reason to begin investing now. Be sure to ask an investment broker what avenues will gain the best compound interest based on the type of investments you choose for your portfolio.

Now that the basics of investing avenues have been outlined, what is the next step? First, decide what type of investments you are willing to explore. There are risks in any investment. In the high-risk category are stocks. During the end of the century and beyond, technology stocks were a hot commodity—volatile to say the least, but many young investors became millionaires practically overnight. However, if retirement is the main objective, stocks will be too risky. Medium-risk investments include mutual funds. As mentioned, mutual funds are a collection of companies, stocks, and bonds. This is a way to invest in many companies at one time. Although the return on investment will not be as high as on stocks, it is a safer, more conservative mechanism to achieve the targeted goal. Many mutual funds will provide a return of 11 percent to over 20 percent per

Table 11–1 Investment Vehicles

Investment Method	Description
Short-term investments	
Savings Accounts	Banking institutions. Mainly offering 2% to 4% per year on the investment
Money Market Funds	Specialized form of mutual funds. Usually pay better interest rates than savings accounts, but lower than certificates of deposit.
Certificate of Deposit (CD)	Specialized deposits made at a bank or other financial institution. Interest rates are higher and may vary depending on the length of the deposit. CDs mature and can be reinvested or cashed with the accumulated interest.
Long-term investments	
Bonds	Available in various forms. Are known as "fixed-income" securities because they generate a fixed income each year. Similar to CDs but they are issued by a government agency.
Stock	A "share" of stock represents a share of ownership in a company. When the value of the company changes, the value of the stock changes.
Mutual Funds	Includes stocks, bonds, and other vehicles. Mutual funds are a collection of investments in one place. Interest rates fluctuate, yet investments can earn over 30% per year.
Retirement Plans	
Individual retirement plan (IRA)	Allows income to be placed into a tax-deferred fund (you do not pay taxes on the income until it is withdrawn).
Roth IRA	A new plan that offers total exemption from federal taxes upon withdrawal. No tax advantages are offered up front, however (cannot be deducted from yearly income taxes). There are income restrictions ($95,000/single; $150,000/married)
401(k)	Offered by employers. Usually the employer matches the funds invested by the employee (if employee invests 10% of salary per month, the employer contributes 10%).

Table 11-1   *Continued*

Investment Method	Description
Retirement Plans	
403(b)	Used in non-profit organizations similar to the 401(k) plan (local and state governments).
Keogh	Specialty IRA. It doubles as a pension plan for self-employed persons. It is limited to $30,000 per year.
Simplified Employee Pension Plan (SEP)	Special kind of Keogh IRA created for small businesses. Employees and employers make contributions.

year. IRAs are another medium-risk to low-risk area where the investment is conservative, provides a tax break (depending on the IRAs chosen), and with regular annual deposits by the investor will help in meeting that retirement goal. In the low-risk category are CDs and bank saving accounts. Low interest rates will not be an advantage unless you are able to make significant deposits each month. No matter what type of avenue you select to begin a retirement portfolio, it will require the expertise of an investment broker to explain how many of these investments work. Some financial investments require a specific amount to open an account and many may require an annual administrative fee. It is wise to take the time to investigate how a retirement plan will work best for you.

What do investment brokers do? Essentially, they are salespersons. They will be the ones to purchase your stocks or mutual funds as requested by you or as recommended to you. Brokers are paid on commission, salary, or both. No matter their compensation, they are experts in investing and in the kind of investments that will suit your needs.

Recently, both novice and experienced investors have been a part of the explosion in **online trading.** This type of investing requires watching the market constantly. There are numerous investment firms that have online trading available for their clients. However, this is not a recommended avenue unless you have the time and you know how online trading works.

Spend Money Wisely

One of the golden rules for investing in a savings mechanism is to "pay yourself first." Many individuals are credit card poor. This means that their hard-earned dollars are spent on trying to pay down credit card balances every month. However, if the interest rate on the card is 18 to 23 percent (which is the average), making that debt disappear will take years. While paying the bills, add one more: yourself. In fact it should be the first bill paid every month. After all, if the money is invested today, it begins to work tomorrow. The interest on that credit card does not.

Many investment experts suggest that a percentage be identified so that regardless of gross or net salary, a predetermined amount has been set aside each month. For those who participate in an employer-paid retirement plan, like a 401(k), 8 percent may be the amount invested by the employee and matched by the employer. Setting a goal of 10 percent to be invested each month will assist in reaching financial goals earlier. Additionally, avoid pitfalls that occur every day to those who want to invest and never seem to accomplish the task:

- Do nothing.
- Start late (better late than never, though).
- Paying down the credit card (better to pay yourself).
- Turn down the retirement plan offered by an employer.

Although each individual or family will have to decide on what is best for them, it is wise to put away as much as possible. This will assure a stable financial future.

INSURANCE COVERAGE FOR DENTAL HYGIENISTS

Along with retirement planning and investments, graduates and practicing professionals are wise to protect themselves by insuring their skills and protecting their profession from possible lawsuits. Life insurance, disability, and liability are three key policies recommended for all practitioners.

During dental hygiene education, many students can protect themselves from possible lawsuits by purchasing liability insurance. Licensed dental hygienists typically will continue with this coverage. **Liability** coverage is essentially **malpractice** insurance. This coverage protects the clinician against financial loss should they be named in a negligence, technical battery, or other lawsuit. Policies can vary among carriers and the practitioner will want to educate him or herself on what will be covered in the policy. Benefits are always limited and will also vary from company to company. For example, an average policy for a dental hygienist may cover up to $3 million per lifetime, with $1 million paid per year per incident as the maximum benefit. The annual premium for such a policy may range from $40 to $90. Upon becoming a member of your professional organization, this type of coverage is available at a group rate.

Disability insurance will assist the professional in monthly income if unable to work for an extended period of time. Suppose the dental hygienist breaks a wrist while skiing or has complications after childbirth and cannot return to work as planned. The disability insurance will provide a certain amount of income (approximately 50 percent of monthly compensation) so that financial obligations can be met. This may help keep bankruptcy in the wings. Additionally, many dental hygienists have been placed on permanent disability due to severe latex allergies and spinal stress disorders due to long-term clinical practice. When this occurs, it prevents the professional from working in a clinical setting, but there are many other positions that can be held by a dental hygienist. Disability premiums range from carrier to carrier. Through professional membership, group rates can be obtained. Due to the high incidence of carpal tunnel syndrome and cumulative stress disorders, many private carriers do not consider the dental hygienist (as they are at a higher risk). This will require some investigation on the part of the practitioner. Many policies require higher premiums or waiting periods before benefits begin, and some may have a threshold on benefits paid over a certain amount of time. Be sure to spend some time with the insurance agent to gain a complete understanding of what the policy entails and to be sure it is right for your lifestyle and the way you practice.

Many states provide disability insurance based on earnings over the last nine months. However, the benefits are far less than what a good disability policy can provide. Dental hygiene salaries can be rather substantial. State disability will not be adequate should you be out of work for an extended period of time.

Life insurance is not always the most pleasant thing to bring up for many individuals. Yet if you do not plan wisely, your family may suffer with unpaid debts and taxes. Life insurance is likely the farthest thing from the minds of graduates who begin their career at a young age. No matter your age, life insurance is something to initiate at the start of this new career. Premiums for life insurance will depend on age. Typically, more mature people pay a higher premium. However, by holding a life insurance policy, you can ensure that your family will be financially stable should their financial support unexpectedly cease. Life insurance policies also vary. There is term life and cash value. Term insurance pays in the event of the purchaser's death. Cash value, or whole life, is a combination of insurance coverage and a savings account. The interest rate on a whole-life policy is typically low compared to other investment options. When investigating the type of life insurance policy right for you and your family, be sure to analyze the options.

Many dental hygienists find they must provide their own health insurance. Unless the practitioner negotiates this benefit through the employer, the entire cost falls to the clinician. Many states have Blue Cross or Blue Shield available to them. Simply making a phone call will provide the necessary information needed to obtain an individual or family policy. Furthermore, some states carry HMO organizations that may offer their coverage to individuals or families not associated with a large company.

Any insurance company will let you know what type of insurance coverage they provide. Not all carriers will provide everything the dental hygienist may need or desire. Thus you may be referred to other insurance carriers. Be prepared to spend some time finding the carrier and policies designed for you.

PROFESSIONAL MEMBERSHIP

As a student, membership in SADHA may have been required (Students of the American Dental Hygienists' Association). Upon graduation and licensure, membership in the professional organization becomes an advantage in many ways. First, insurance companies offer group rates to organizations. Many find that this benefit suits their financial plan, since many premiums are expensive. The ADHA offers all types of insurance coverage to its members. In addition to disability, liability, life, and major medical, home and auto insurance can also be purchased through ADHA. However, the policy limitations may differ from a private carrier. The most common variations are the length of benefits, maximum of benefits, deductible, and waiting period. Again, it is worthwhile to compare policies.

Insurance is only one benefit of membership, and it is a tangible benefits. Intangible benefits are more numerous and may be of more value than the tangible benefits. Undoubtedly, dental hygiene students have been introduced to their professional organization at some level: national, state, or local. The membership fee is relatively inexpensive for the many benefits provided. Essentially, membership is approximately the compensation received by the clinician for one day's work—easy enough to come by. Intangible benefits include networking with other professionals, participating in legislative issues, mentoring, representing the local component to the national organization, educational support, continuing education, and research avenues. The benefits are numerous, both tangible and intangible. It is wise for new licentiates to maintain their membership while maintaining their license.

SELF-CARE

Cumulative trauma disorder (CTD) is defined as musculoskeletal disorders that can result from the body's inability to heal itself from the long-term effects of repetitive motion, exposure to vibration, and mechanical stress. According to the U.S. Bureau of Labor Statistics, CTD is the fastest growing occupational disorder. The dental hygiene field remains among the top ten occupations for CTD. Although many aspects of dental hygiene have seen modification to reduce stress disorders, students and practitioners will want to remain active and healthy to increase career longevity. No longer do clinicians grasp small diametered instruments; there is a diverse selection of handles that make it easier for the clinician to decrease muscle fatigue in the hands and wrists. Operator chairs are now ergonomically designed to provide better lower back support and a place to rest the forearm. Ultrasonic units and slow speed handpieces have been designed specifically to decrease the weight and vibrations placed on the practitioner's arms and wrists.

Body positioning in relation to the patient plays an important part in posture while scaling and root planing all day long. Exercise is a priority for those who want to ensure the length of their career. Clinicians should avoid slouching over the patient for direct vision and should work more with the mirror, eliminating the stress placed on the spine. Many students tend to cross their ankles or legs while working in the seven o'clock position. This puts stress on the spine and may create muscle fatigue on the lower back, as the body must lean slightly to maintain an upright position. Patients are willing to comply so that the clinician gains better access. Ask the patient to turn his or her head, tilt upward, tilt downward, or whatever it takes to decrease the stress on your body. Some patients are not able to comply due to their own medical or physical condition. However, this is not likely to happen every day in private practice, unless the practitioner is employed with a facility caring for such patients. For these patients, practitioners will have to compensate their positioning for the patient.

In order to increase career longevity, the dental hygienist must place his or her health first. This includes diet and exercise. A balanced diet full of nutritious foods will help you to avoid the common cold, influenza, and other seasonal, communicable diseases that occur in patients seen every day all year long. Water consumption remains the number one objective in the best of diets. Keep the body hydrated, consume fruits and vegetables more frequently than starchy items. Limit saturated fats and sugars. By doing so, body weight can be managed, body fat can be managed, and energy levels will increase. A balanced diet can assist in protection from harmful systemic diseases.

Exercise plays an important role in maintaining a healthy posture through strengthening the muscles that surround the skeletal system. For many, membership in a health club is the only thing that will motivate them to exercise. For others, taking advantage of the outdoors through various activities keeps them active. The American College of Sports Medicine recommends that exercise be done at least 30 minutes every day. Other sources may recommend 4 to 5 times per week. Exercise comes in various forms; however, just walking will provide activity and improved health. An activity plan may also require some time management in order to fit it into a busy schedule. Lunch breaks are a great opportunity to walk for 30 minutes. Participating in organized functions like walk-a-thons and races is another way to spend some time outside of those operatory walls.

No matter the choice of activity to incorporate into your lifestyle, the benefits will be seen in a variety of ways.

- Weight loss/increased muscle tone
- Increased energy/healthier food choices
- Decreased depression/increased social interaction
- Decreased illness

By making subtle changes in lifestyle, many practitioners will realize career longevity. Furthermore, many of the CTDs are decreased, thus decreasing the possibility of surgical procedures.

Another preventative measure for muscle and skeletal fatigue is massage therapy. This may be one of the most popular and successful avenues in prevention of stress disorders. Massage therapy on a regular basis aids not only in relaxing tight muscles around the skeletal system, but also in relaxing the mind. It allows the practitioner some quiet time that helps to alleviate the mental and physical stresses of dental hygiene procedures. Many physicians advocate the value of including massage therapy in your preventive care routine. There are dental practices that have begun to include a massage therapist in their benefits for employees. The dentist will have the massage therapist visit the practice once a month and provide 15-minute sessions to employees. This assists in the overall wellness of staff members. Massage therapy can be scheduled as easily as a hair appointment and is a relatively inexpensive preventive measure that can add to career longevity. Millions of dollars are lost annually by dental practitioners due to CTDs and related pain. Take proactive measures to ensure that it does not happen to you or your family.

For those who are experiencing some kind of CTD or other condition, you are not alone. There are many who currently experience some kind of pain. Myofacial pain, myalgia, carpal tunnel, and neck and shoulder problems are among a few. Carol Coady, RDH, is one dental hygienist who has dealt with occupational pain and developed the Hygienists' Pain Network. Coady resides in northern California and remains involved with allied organizations that target individuals dealing with chronic pain. Professionals can exchange and share information that helps them deal with occupational pain or provides information on resources for professional care. For those interested in communicating with other professionals to share experiences or to find out how they have dealt with an occupational stress disorder, visit *www.cdha.org* and click on the phrase "occupational pain." Additionally, many articles can be found on *www.rdh.net*. This and related sites may provide answers to questions on preventing cumulative stress disorders.

No matter the type of exercise or activity you choose, a balanced diet is essential for a healthy lifestyle. Numerous preventive measures must be employed, and the dental hygienist will want to make a concerted effort to lengthen the life of his or her chosen profession. The cost of a dental hygiene education can be abruptly interrupted, without the proper fitness routine. Each professional will want to take the time to organize his or her career so as to benefit from the efforts placed into obtaining educational and career goals. The key to career longevity is prevention of cumulative stress disorders.

Summary

Upon graduation, financial planning is the first step to ensure that retirement goals are realized. Developing financial goals and seeking expert advice will assist in outlining a financial plan best suited to your specific needs. A diverse portfolio is one of the best ways to increase self-wealth. There are numerous avenues available for investments, and it will take some research to select the best investments to meet your retirement goals. Investments range from high-risk to low-risk. Each individual and family will want to select investments wisely.

Insurance coverage for dental hygienists is recommended. Disability insurance provides benefits if you are unable to work due to long-term illness, medical complications, or accident. Liability or malpractice insurance provides benefits in the event of lawsuits in which the dental hygienist is named. There are limitations on the amount of benefits provided per year and per lifetime. Life insurance will provide for those family members who remain in the event of an untimely death. Premiums for all types of insurance policies vary, as do the companies who offer them. Membership in your professional organization will assist in tangible and intangible benefits. Career longevity will depend on how well the practitioner maintains his or her health. Avoidance of musculoskeletal disorders must be a priority if the dental hygienist plans on a long professional career. Preventive measures include ergonomically designed instruments and equipment, as well as a balanced diet and regular exercise.

SELF-TEST

1. Describe the differences between a stock and a mutual fund.
2. Why are mutual funds a better investment than a CD from your local bank?
3. What is a diverse portfolio?
4. Obtain a copy of the local newspaper and locate the stock report. Select five companies and find out how much a share has increased or decreased in value. After three days, locate the same five companies to see the change in value. For example, locate Microsoft, General Motors, Walmart, Amazon.com, and Home Depot.
5. Explain why the dental hygienist will want to purchase disability insurance.
6. List some of the benefits of a healthy lifestyle.

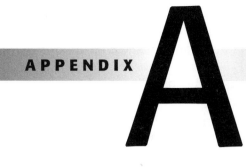

Code of Ethics of the American Dental Hygienists' Association

1. PREAMBLE

As dental hygienists, we are a community of professionals devoted to the prevention of disease and the promotion and improvement of the public's health. We are preventive oral health professionals who provide educational, clinical, and therapeutic services to the public. We strive to live meaningful, productive, satisfying lives that simultaneously serve us, our profession, our society, and the world. Our actions, behaviors, and attitudes are consistent with our commitment to public service. We endorse and incorporate the Code into our daily lives.

2. PURPOSE

The purpose of a professional code of ethics is to achieve high levels of ethical consciousness, decision making, and practice by the members of the profession. Specific objectives of the Dental Hygiene Code of Ethics are

- to increase our professional and ethical consciousness and sense of ethical responsibility.
- to lead us to recognize ethical issues and choices and to guide us in making more informed ethical decisions.
- to establish a standard for professional judgment and conduct.
- to provide a statement of the ethical behavior the public can expect from us.

The Dental Hygiene Code of Ethics is meant to influence us throughout our careers. It stimulates our continuing study of ethical issues and challenges us to explore our ethical responsibilities. The Code establishes concise standards of behavior to guide the public's expectations of our profession and supports dental hygiene practice, laws and regulations. By holding ourselves accountable to meeting the standards stated in the Code, we enhance the public's trust on which our professional privilege and status are founded.

3. Key Concepts

Our beliefs, principles, values and ethics are concepts reflected in the Code. They are the essential elements of our comprehensive and definitive code of ethics, and are interrelated and mutually dependent.

4. Basic Beliefs

We recognize the importance of the following beliefs that guide our practice and provide context for our ethics:

- The services we provide contribute to the health and well being of society.
- Our education and licensure qualify us to serve the public by preventing and treating oral disease and helping individuals achieve and maintain optimal health.
- Individuals have intrinsic worth, are responsible for their own health, and are entitled to make choices regarding their health.
- Dental hygiene care is an essential component of overall health care and we function interdependently with other health care providers.
- All people should have access to health care, including oral health care.
- We are individually responsible for our actions and the quality of care we provide.

These fundamental principles, universal concepts and general laws of conduct provide the foundation for our ethics.

Universality

The principle of universality expects that, if one individual judges an action to be right or wrong in a given situation, other people considering the same action in the same situation would make the same judgment.

Complementarity

The principle of complementarity recognizes the existence of an obligation to justice and basic human rights. In all relationships, it requires considering the values and perspectives of others before making decisions or taking actions affecting them.

Ethics

Ethics are the general standards of right and wrong that guide behavior within society. As generally accepted actions, they can be judged by determining the extent to which they promote good and minimize harm. Ethics compel us to engage in health promotion/disease prevention activities.

Community

This principle expresses our concern for the bond between individuals, the community, and society in general. It leads us to preserve natural resources and inspires us to show concern for the global environment.

Responsibility

Responsibility is central to our ethics. We recognize that there are guidelines for making ethical choices and accept responsibility for knowing and applying them. We accept the consequences of our actions or the failure to act and are willing to make ethical choices and publicly affirm them.

6. Core Values

We acknowledge these values as general for our choices and actions.

Individual Autonomy and Respect for Human Beings

People have the right to be treated with respect. They have the right to informed consent prior to treatment, and they have the right to full disclosure of all relevant information so that they can make informed choices about their care.

Confidentiality

We respect the confidentiality of client information and relationships as a demonstration of the value we place on individual autonomy. We acknowledge our obligation to justify any violation of a confidence.

Societal Trust

We value client trust and understand that public trust in our profession is based on our actions and behavior.

Nonmaleficence

We accept our fundamental obligation to provide services in a manner that protects all clients and minimizes harm to them and others involved in their treatment.

Beneficence

We have a primary role in promoting the well being of individuals and the public by engaging in health promotion/disease prevention activities.

Justice and Fairness

We value justice and support the fair and equitable distribution of health care resources. We believe all people should have access to high-quality, affordable oral healthcare.

Veracity

We accept our obligation to tell the truth and expect that others will do the same. We value self-knowledge and seek truth and honesty in all relationships.

7. STANDARDS OF PROFESSIONAL RESPONSIBILITY

We are obligated to practice our profession in a manner that supports our purpose, beliefs, and values in accordance with the fundamental principles that support our ethics. We acknowledge the following responsibilities:

To Ourselves as Individuals . . .

- Avoid self-deception, and continually strive for knowledge and personal growth.
- Establish and maintain a lifestyle that supports optimal health.
- Create a safe work environment.
- Assert our own interests in ways that are fair and equitable.
- Seek the advice and counsel of others when challenged with ethical dilemmas.
- Have realistic expectations of ourselves and recognize our limitations.

To Ourselves as Professionals . . .

- Enhance professional competencies through continuous learning in order to practice according to high standards of care.
- Support dental hygiene peer-review systems and quality-assurance measures.
- Develop collaborative professional relationships and exchange knowledge to enhance our own lifelong professional development.

To Family and Friends . . .

- Support the efforts of others to establish and maintain healthy lifestyles and respect the rights of friends and family.

To Clients . . .

- Provide oral health care utilizing high levels of professional knowledge, judgment, and skill.
- Maintain a work environment that minimizes the risk of harm.
- Serve all clients without discrimination and avoid action toward any individual or group that may be interpreted as discriminatory.
- Hold professional client relationships confidential.

- Communicate with clients in a respectful manner.
- Promote ethical behavior and high standards of care by all dental hygienists.
- Serve as an advocate for the welfare of clients.
- Provide clients with the information necessary to make informed decisions about their oral health and encourage their full participation in treatment decisions and goals.
- Refer clients to other healthcare providers when their needs are beyond our ability or scope of practice.
- Educate clients about high-quality oral health care.

To Colleagues . . .

- Conduct professional activities and programs, and develop relationships in ways that are honest, responsible, and appropriately open and candid.
- Encourage a work environment that promotes individual professional growth and development.
- Collaborate with others to create a work environment that minimizes risk to the personal health and safety of our colleagues.
- Manage conflicts constructively.
- Support the efforts of other dental hygienists to communicate the dental hygiene philosophy and preventive oral care.
- Inform other health care professionals about the relationship between general and oral health.
- Promote human relationships that are mutually beneficial, including those with other health care professionals.

To Employees and Employers . . .

- Conduct professional activities and programs, and develop relationships in ways that are honest, responsible, open, and candid.
- Manage conflicts constructively.
- Support the right of our employees and employers to work in an environment that promotes wellness.
- Respect the employment rights of our employers and employees.

To the Dental Hygiene Profession . . .

- Participate in the development and advancement of our profession.
- Avoid conflicts of interest and declare them when they occur.

- Seek opportunities to increase public awareness and understanding of oral health practices.
- Act in ways that bring credit to our profession while demonstrating appropriate respect for colleagues in other professions.
- Contribute time, talent, and financial resources to support and promote our profession.
- Promote a positive image for our profession.
- Promote a framework for professional education that develops dental hygiene competencies to meet the oral and overall health needs of the public.

To the Community and Society . . .

- Recognize and uphold the laws and regulations governing our profession.
- Document and report inappropriate, inadequate, or substandard care and/or illegal activities by an health care provider, to the responsible authorities.
- Use peer review as a mechanism for identifying inappropriate, inadequate, or substandard care provided by dental hygienists.
- Comply with local, state, and federal statutes that promote public health and safety.
- Develop support systems and quality-assurance programs in the workplace to assist dental hygienist in providing the appropriate standard of care.
- Promote access to dental hygiene services for all, supporting justice and fairness in the distribution of healthcare resources.
- Act consistently with the ethics of the global scientific community of which our profession is a part.
- Create a healthful workplace ecosystem to support a healthy environment.
- Recognize and uphold our obligation to provide pro bono service.

To Scientific Investigation . . .

We accept responsibility for conducting research according to the fundamental principles underlying our ethical beliefs in compliance with universal codes, governmental standards, and professional guidelines for the care and management of experimental subjects. We acknowledge our ethical obligations to the scientific community:

- Conduct research that contributes knowledge that is valid and useful to our clients and society.
- Use research methods that meet accepted scientific standards.
- Use research resources appropriately.
- Systematically review and justify research in progress to insure the most favorable benefit-to-risk ratio to research subjects.
- Submit all proposals involving human subjects to an appropriate human subject review committee.
- Secure appropriate institutional committee approval for the conduct of research involving animals.
- Obtain informed consent from human subjects participating in research that is based on specification published in Title 21 Code of Federal Regulations Part 46.
- Respect the confidentiality and privacy of data.
- Seek opportunities to advance dental hygiene knowledge through research by providing financial, human, and technical resources whenever possible.
- Report research results in a timely manner.
- Report research findings completely and honestly, drawing only those conclusions that are supported by the data presented.
- Report the names of investigators fairly and accurately.
- Interpret the research and the research of others accurately and objectively, drawing conclusions that are supported by the data presented and seeking clarity when uncertain.
- Critically evaluate research methods and results before applying new theory and technology in practice.
- Be knowledgeable concerning currently accepted preventive and therapeutic methods, products, and technology and their application to our practice.

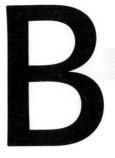

Regional Board
Exam Agencies

Central Regional Dental Testing Service, Inc. (CRDTS)

Address: 1725 Gage Blvd.
          Topeka, KS 66604

Phone: (931) 273–0830

Web site: *www.crdts.org*

Northeast Regional Board of Dental Examiners, Inc. (NERB)

Address: 8484 Georgia Ave., Suite 900
          Silver Springs, MD 20910

Phone: (301) 563–3300

Web site: *www.nerb.org*

Note: October 2000. Information is subject to change.

Southern Regional Testing Agency, Inc. (SRTA)

Address:	Ocean Plaza Corp. Center
	303 34th Street, Suite 7
	Virgina Beach, VA 23451
Phone:	(575) 428–1003
Web site:	*www.srta.org*

Western Regional Examining Board (WREB)

Address:	9201 North 25th Ave., Suite 185
	Phoenix, AZ 85021
Phone:	(602) 944–3315
Web site:	*www. werb.org*

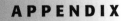

C

State Participation in Board Exams

State	CRTS	NERB	SRBA	WREB	Individual
Alabama					x
Arkansas			x		
Arizona				x	
California					x
Colorado	x				
Connecticut		x			
Delaware					x
Florida					x
Georgia			x		
Hawaii					x
Idaho				x	
Illinois	x	x			
Indiana					x
Iowa	x				
Kansas	x				
Kentucky			x		

(*continued*)

State	CRTS	NERB	SRBA	WREB	Individual
Louisiana					x
Maine		x			
Maryland		x			
Massachusetts		x			
Michigan		x			
Minnesota	x				
Mississippi					x
Missouri	x				
Montana				x	
Nebraska	x				
Nevada					x
New Hampshire		x			
New Jersey		x			
New Mexico				x	
New York		x			
North Carolina					x
North Dakota	x				
Ohio		x			
Oklahoma				x	
Oregon				x	
Pennsylvania		x			
Rhode Island		x			
South Carolina	x				x
South Dakota	x				
Tennessee			x		
Texas				x	
Utah				x	
Vermont		x			
Virginia		x			
Washington				x	
Washington, DC		x			
West Virginia		x			
Wisconsin	x				
Wyoming	x				

Source: www.adha.org; www.crdts.org; www.nerb.org; www.crta.org; www.wreb.org on October 19, 2000.
Note: A state may not participate in a regional board, yet accept it.

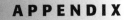

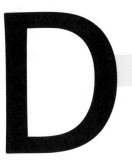

Permitted Dental Hygiene Functions and Levels of Supervision

ADHA Practice Act Overview Chart of Permitted Functions and Supervision Levels by State

	AL	AK	AZ	AR	CA	CO	CT	DE	DC	FL	GA
Prophylaxis	P	N	N	P/N	N/U	N/U	N/U	N	N	N	P
X-rays	P	N	N	P	N/U	N	N/U	N	N	N	P
Local Anesthesia		P	P	P	P	P					
Topical Anesthesia	P	N	N	P	N/U	N/U	N/U	N	N	N	P
Fluoride	P	N	N	P	N/U	N/U	N/U	N	N	N	P
Pit/Fissure Sealants	P	N	N	P	N/U	N/U	N/U	N	P	P	P
Root Planing	P	N	N	P	N/U	N	N/U	N	N	P	P
Soft Tissue Curettage	P	N	N	P	P	N/U		N		P	P
Administer N^2O		P	P	P	P	P					
Study Cast Impressions	P	N	N	P	N/U	N	N/U	N	P	N	P
Place Perio Dressings	P	N	P		N/U	N	N/U	N	P	N	P
Remove Perio Dressing	P	N	P	P	N/U	N	N/U	N	P	N	P
Place Sutures		N	N/P								
Remove Sutures	P	N	N	P	N/U	N	N/U	N	P	N	P
Apply Cavity—Liners & Bases	P	P	N			N				P	
Place Temporary Restorations	P	N	N	P	N/U	N		N	P	N	P
Remove Temporary Restorations	P	N	N	P	N/U	N		N	P	N	
Place Amalgam Restorations						N					P
Carve Amalgam Restorations					P	N					P
Finish Amalgam Restorations						N					
Polish Amalgram Restorations	P	N	N	P	N/U	N	N/U	N	N	N	P
Place & Finish—Composite Resin Silicate Restore						N					

Key: P = Physical presence of dentist is required

    N = Physical presence of dentist is not required

    U = Physical presence not required. No prior authorization by dentist required but there may be requirement for type of cooperative arrangement with a dentist(s). Some states require experience or special education by RDH.

    l = Where two letters are present in a box the first indicates the supervision level in the private dental office. The second indicates the supervision level in other settings such as independent dental practice, long-term facilities, hospitals, etc. on nonambulatory patients.

Source: Copyright American Dental Hygienists' Association. Reprinted by permission.

HI	ID	IL	IN	IA	KS	KY	LA	ME	MD	MA	MI	MN	MS
P/N	N	P/N	P/U	N	N	P	P/N	N	P/N	N	N/U	N	P/N
P/N	N	P/N	P	N	N	P	P/N	N	P/N	N	N	N	P/N
P	P	P		P	P		P	P				P	
P/N	N	P/N	P	N	N	P	P/N	N	P/N	N	N	N	
P/N	N	P/N	P	N	N	P	P/N	N	P/N	N	N	N	P
P/N	N	P/N	P	N	N	P	P/N	N	P/N	N	N	N	P
P/N	N	P/N	P	N	N	P	P/N	N	P/N	N	N	N	P
P/N		P/N		N	N	P		N		N	P	N	P
	P	P		P	N							P	
P/N	P	P/N	P	N	N	P	P	N	P	N	N	N	P
P/N			P	N	N	P		P	P/N	N	N	N	P
P/N	N	P/N	P	N	N	P	P/N	N	P/N	N	N	N	P
P/N													
P/N	N	P/N	P	N	N	P	P/N	N	P/N	N	N	N	P
	P		P	N		P					N	N	
P/N	N	P/N	P	N	N	P	P	N	P	N		N	P
	N	P/N	P	N	N	P	P			P		N	P
			P			P				P			
			P			P							
			P			P							
P/N	N	P/N	P	N	N	P	P	N	P	N	N	N	P
			P			P							

(*continued*)

ADHA Practice Act Overview Chart of Permitted Functions and Supervision Levels by State (*continued*)

	MO	MT	NE	NV	NH	NJ	NM	NY	NC	ND	OH
Prophylaxis	N	N	N	N	N	P/N	N	N	P	N	N
X-rays	N	N	N	N	N	P/N	N	N	P	N	N
Local Anesthesia	P	P	P	P		P					
Topical Anesthesia	N	N	N	N	N	P/N	N	N	P	N	N
Fluoride	N	N	N	N	N	P/N	N	N	P	N	N
Pit/Fissure Sealants	N	N	N	N	N	P	N	N	P	N	P
Root Planing	N	N	N	P	N	P/N	N	N	P	N	P
Soft Tissue Curettage	N	N	N	P		P/N	N			N	P
Administer N^{2}O	P			P							
Study Cast Impressions	N	N	N	N	N	P	N	P	P	P	N
Place Perio Dressings	P	N	N	N		P		P		P	P
Remove Perio Dressing	P	N	N	N	N	P	N	P	P	P	N
Place Sutures											
Remove Sutures	P	N	N	N	N	P		P	P	P	P
Apply Cavity—Liners & Bases									P		P
Place Temporary Restorations	N	N	N	N		P	N	P	P	P	P
Remove Temporary Restorations	N	N	N	N		P	N	P	P	P	P
Place Amalgam Restorations						P					P
Carve Amalgam Restorations											P
Finish Amalgam Restorations											P
Polish Amalgram Restorations	P/N	N	N	N	N	P	N	N	P	P	P
Place & Finish—Composite Resin Silicate Restore											P

Key: P = Physical presence of dentist is required

N = Physical presence of dentist is not required

U = Physical presence not required. No prior authorization by dentist required but there may be requirement for type of cooperative arrangement with a dentist(s). Some states require experience or special education by RDH.

l = Where two letters are present in a box the first indicates the supervision level in the private dental office. The second indicates the supervision level in other settings such as independent dental practice, long-term facilities, hospitals, etc. on nonambulatory patients.

Source: Copyright American Dental Hygienists' Association. Reprinted by permission.

OK	OR	PA	RI	SC	SD	TN	TX	UT	VT	VA	WA	WV	WI	WY
N	N/U	P/N	N	P/N	N	N	N	N	N	P	N/U	P	N/U	N
N	N/U	P/N	N	P	P	N	N	N	N	P	N	P	N	N
P	N			P	P			P	P		P		P	P
N	N/U	P/N	N	P	P	P	N	N	N	P	N	P	N	N
N	N/U	P/N	N	P/N	P	P	N	N	N	P	N/U	P	N	N
N	N	P/N	N	P/N	N	P	N	N	N	P	N	P	N	P
N	N/U	P/N	N	P/N	P	P	N	N	N	P	N/U	P	N	N
P	N/U				P	P		N			P/U			
P	P				P	P		P			P			
N	N/U	P	P	P		P	N	N	N	P	N	P	N	N
N	N/U		P				N	N	N	P	P	P	N	P
N	N/U		P	P	P	P	N	N	N	P	P	P	N	P
								N						
N	N/U	P	P	P		P	N	N	N	P	P	P	N	N
		P	P								P			
N	N/U		P			P	N	N	N		P			N
N			P			P	N	N	N					
						P				P	P			P
											P			P
									N		P			P
N	N/U	P	P	P	N	P	N	N	N	P	N	P	N	N
											P			P

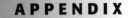

E

Components of a Marketing Plan (Alternative Practice)

I. **Develop an action plan**
   A. Review goals and objectives
      1. research the existing market
      2. conduct a survey (patients, employees)
      3. identify the identity of the practice (what makes the practice unique)
   B. Develop a marketing strategy (how to achieve the goals)
      1. are staff members supportive?
   C. Get involved with the community (activities, events, sponsorships)
   D. Develop public relations (media releases or exposure)
   E. Implement the plan
   F. Reevaluate periodically for effectiveness or modification
II. **Marketing will assist in numerous ways**
   A. Attracting new patients or patient contacts
      1. educating
      2. loyalty

      B. Communicate
         1. who you are
         2. what you do
         3. assist in how others perceive you and the practice
      C. Increase cash flow
         1. increased production (increase in patients)
         2. increase the referral base
         3. create good will with others in the community
      D. Create and enhance the image of the practice and professional
         1. quality service
         2. quality staff

III. What marketing is unable to achieve
      A. Hide or disguise poor quality service
         1. compensate for insensitive staff members/inefficiency
         2. hide unsanitary conditions or maintenance of the practice/ equipment

Those who choose to advance into alternative practice will find it necessary to create a marketing and public relations plan. Seeking advice from a management consultant may benefit the dental hygiene professional.

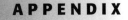

F

Interview Tips: The Basics

- Be certain of the time and place of the interview.
- Arrive at least 15 minutes early for the interview.
- Bring a pen and note book; take notes of important information learned from the interview.
- Remember the interviewer's name.
- Be proactive and shake hands.
- Dress appropriately for the job.
- Do not smoke or chew gum.
- Do not monopolize the interviewer's time; share in the conversation.
- Learn as much about the business as you can.
- Get comfortable talking about your own skills and abilities. Recognize your strengths and weaknesses.
- Be yourself. Answer questions honestly, not how you think they want them answered.
- Be prepared to ask about the duties of the position and how you are capable of performing those duties.
- Follow up on the interview. A thank-you note is appropriate for jobs in which you are very interested.

G

Sample Interview Questions

Questions from the employer

- May I see your resume?
- What can I do for you?
- Why are you interested in joining our office?
- What do you feel qualifies you for this position?
- What can you do for us?
- Tell me about your experience.

Questions regarding motivation

- Why do you want to change jobs?
- What caused you to enter this field?
- What part of your career interests you the most?

Questions regarding education

- Describe your education for me.
- What courses did you like the best and least, and why?
- What kinds of community activities were included?

Questions regarding pay

- What kind of salary are you seeking?
- What is the minimum pay you will accept?
- What did you receive at your last position?
- We can't pay the salary you are asking for right now. Would you be willing to start lower and work up to that figure?
- What do you expect to be earning in five years?

Questions from the potential employee

- How long have you been in practice?
- How many patients are seen per day?
- How many dental hygienists are employed in your office?
- What is the size of your staff?
- Are there office policy manuals?

Questions regarding motivation

- How long has your staff been with you?
- Why did the last dental hygienist leave?
- How many hygiene days would you prefer?
- What is your philosophy regarding preventive care?
- How often do your refer patients to the specialist?

Questions regarding education

- Where did you attend dental school?
- How often does the staff attend continuing education courses?
- Are continuing education courses a benefit for all employees?
- What part of dentistry interests you the most?

Questions regarding experience

- Why are you seeking a dental hygienist? (another dental hygienist?)
- What duties do you expect from your dental hygienist?
- Who generally makes the decisions for the practice?
- Who is my immediate supervisor?
- How are conflicts handled in the office (employees/patients)?

Questions regarding pay

- What is the average salary for dental hygienists in your office?
- What is the minimum/maximum you will pay?

- How are dental hygienists compensated in your practice? (daily, commission, hourly)
- What other benefits do you currently provide for employees? (medical, dental, profit sharing, uniforms, continuing education)
- How often are salaries reviewed?
- Are you willing to negotiate benefits at a later date?

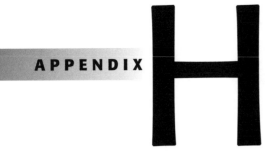
Internet Resources

www.adha.org   American Dental Hygienists' Association

www.ada.org   American Dental Association
- National Board Dental Hygiene Examination

www.aarp.org   American Association of Retired People

www.eeoc.gov   Equal Employment Opportunity Commission (EEOC)

www.osha.gov   Occupational Safety and Health Administration

www.cdc.gov   Center for Disease Control
- Violence in the workplace

www.hcfa.gov   Health Care Financing Administration
- Medicaid
- Medicare
- SCHIP

www.childabuse.org   Prevent Child Abuse America

www.netscape.com   Investing basics

- Stocks
- Mutual Funds
- Selecting a broker
- Stretching the life of your IRA
- Do-it-yourself retirement plans

www.gag.org (2000)   "Negotiate that contract"

www.geekeducation.com (2000)   "How to negotiate (and get what you want)" by Kimberly Wandel

www.mcn.org (2000)   "How to build a Team"

www.gmu.edu (2000)   "Characteristics of an effective team"

www.anita-jupp.nas.net   Anita Jupp & Company, Dental Practice Management

www.a-d-h.com   ADH Practice Solutions with Linda Miles

www.tramtechnology.co.uk (2000)   The Basics of Team Building

www.mnworkforcecenter.org (2000)   Creative Job Search: Dress and Grooming for Job Success.

- Job success skills
- Employment application
- Employment interviews
- Cover letter and thank-you notes
- The job search

Note: Internet sites may change. Searching the Internet via keywords is another option for obtaining information.

Glossary

Abandon: to end a patient-provider relationship; terminate treatment or refrain from seeing the patient.

Access to care: individual's ability to obtain timely personal health (and dental) care; access to care is hindered by financial resources, location of providers, distance and transportation problems, and sociological barriers.

Accounts receivable: accounts, usually incurred by patients, whereby the money is owed to the practice for services received.

Accreditation: process by which standards are guaranteed.

Act utilitarian: a utilitarian who is concerned with individual acts.

Advanced Appointment System: a system that allows the patient to obtain an appointment in the distance future: 3 months, six months.

Assault: threatening to harm an individual; a type of tort or civil wrong. Technical assault is no intention of harming; similar to technical battery.

Authoritative management: occurs when the dentist or one person makes all the decisions for the practice.

Autonomy: self-determination; a core value or ethical principle found in a code of ethics; necessary for informed consent and patient as partner in treatment.

Battery: touching an individual with the intention to harm; a type of tort or civil wrong. Technical battery is no intention of harming, but actually touching without permission; similar to technical assault.

Beneficence: doing what will benefit the patient; a core value or ethical principle found in a code of ethics.

Benefits: Anything over and above salary and provided by the employer at no cost to the employee.

Capitation: a flatfee provided to a dentist or provider by a third party or insurance payor regardless of the dental procedures performed based on the number of consumers enrolled on the plan.

Case law: common law; law determined by court judgments, not by legislation.

Cash flow: a steady flow of revenue or income for services provided.

Child abuse: any act that endangers or impairs a child's physical or emotional health or development.

Civil law: one of two types of statutory law; concerns offenses or wrongful acts against an individual person, property, or reputation; includes tort and contract law; seeks to compensate the victim.

Common law: case law; law determined by court judgments, not by legislation.

Compound interest: interest paid on both the principal and the accumulated interest

Confidentiality: avoidance of disseminating or revealing any personal or private information about the patient; a core value or ethical principle found in a code of ethics; also, duty to the patient bound by law.

Consequential theory: type of normative ethics that judges an action as right or wrong by the consequences; utilitarianism is the best known consequentialist theory.

Contracts: legal agreements; part of civil law; can be either implied or expressed.

Cost of Living: an index that correlates with increases in standards of living. How much does it cost to maintain a standard of life? Increases may range from 3 to 5% each year based on increases for all products purchased by consumers.

Credentials: qualifications that entitle an individual to license, authority, etc.

Criminal law: one of two types of statutory law; concerns offenses against society; seeks to punish the offender through loss of life or liberty, or through fines.

Crosstraining: implies that each member in the office has been trained to perform duties of other staff members. Limitations will apply for licensed personnel.

Decision making: process utilizing critical thinking skills to arrive at a judgment or conclusion.

Defamation: making false statements that harms an individual's reputation; can be either libel (written) or slander (verbal); involves communication to a third person; a type of tort or civil wrong.

Dental Health Maintenance Organization: an organization designed to promote the prevention of oral disease by enabling consumers to enroll for an annual fee and then to have access to all procedures without having to pay an additional fee.

Dental Hygiene Diagnosis: the act of identifying an actual or potential human need deficit related to oral health or disease that the dental hygienist is educated and licensed to treat.

Deontology: branch of normative ethics that emphasizes duties.

Dilemma: situation necessitating a choice between two equal, especially undesirable, alternatives.

Direct approach: a system where staff members of the dental office will directly contact patients to schedule periodic examination and dental hygiene appointments.

Disability: any physical, condition, injury or illness that disables a person to perform duties that are employment related in a normal fashion.

Distributive justice: fairly distribution or allocation of resources.

Domestic violence: violence that occurs in the home or within the family; spouse abuse, wife battering, or abusing an individual having an intimate contact.

Duty: obligation; action that ought to be done regardless of consequences.

Efficacy: to produce effects or intended results

Elderly abuse: physical or sexual abuse, emotional confinement, passive neglect, willful deprivation, and financial exploitation.

Ethical dilemma: conflict between moral obligations that are difficult to reconcile.

Ethics: discipline consisting of thoughts and ideas about morality; judging actions right or wrong.

Evaluations: review of employee performance based on job descriptions and/ or determination of the worth or value of an employee by an employer or supervisor

Fidelity: faithful to promises and obligations; a core value or ethical principle found in a code of ethics; closely related to veracity, trust, and confidentiality.

Free-rein management: occurs when no one particular person is the authority figure in the practice.

Health maintenance organization (HMO): managed care; system of health care delivery that controls utilization and costs of service to deliver cost-effective care.

Huddle: a daily meeting that occurs each morning or other agreed upon time, wherein the entire staff reviews the daily schedule and patient charts.

Indirect approach: a system that uses other methods of contacting patients for future appointments: postcards, mailers, notices.

Informed consent: patient's acceptance (or refusal) of a line of treatment based on the information provided by a health care provider; an ethical and legal consideration.

Jurisprudence: science or philosophy of law.

Justice: fairness and impartiality; a core value or ethical principle found in a code of ethics.

Liability: the state of being liable to another party (providing a service that has been promised)

Libel: written or published defamation; one of two types of defamation, the other being slander (verbal).

Life Insurance: insurance in which a stipulated sum of money is paid to a named beneficiary or beneficiaries at the death of the insured.

Mail System: a system that uses regular mail delivery to notify consumers of a needed dental visit. Postcards are typically used and the patient becomes responsible to follow through with obtaining the appointment.

Malpractice: professional negligence; not performing standard of care and harm results; part of tort law, civil law.

Managed care: health maintenance organization (HMO); system of health care delivery that controls utilization and costs of service to deliver cost-effective care.

Marketing: a social and managerial process by which individuals and groups obtain what they need through exchange of products or services that have value.

Medicaid: federal government health care assistance, enacted by each state, for indigent or low-income individuals.

Medicare: federal government health care assistance for individuals 65 years or older; largest health insurance program in United States.

Merit: recognition of worth or value

Negligence: not performing or measuring up to the standards of a reasonable and prudent person and harm results; see malpractice and professional negligence.

Nonmaleficence: to do no harm to others; a core value or ethical principle found in a code of ethics.

Normative ethics: metaethics; branch of ethics which recommends specific actions as right and justified.

Online Trading: the act of investing, buying or selling stocks, mutuals funds or notes, using an Internet source.

Overhead: the amount (in money or finances) that it costs to operate a business.

Parentalism: paternalism; acting like a father or parent that knows what is best for the patient; making a decision for the patient.

Participatory management: occurs when all staff members participate in the decision-making process for the practice.

Paternalism: parentalism; acting like a father or parent that knows what is best for the patient; making a decision for the patient.

Patients' bill of rights: rights of a patient guaranteed by the provider, the institution providing services, or the government; duties of the provider the patient can expect.

Policy manuals: each practice will develop manuals that assist all personnel in understanding the rules, regulations, and duties that pertain to the daily operations of the practice. Manuals can be developed for numerous categories.

Portfolio: a collection of papers, manuscripts, drawings; anything pertinent to a specific assignment, job or class.

Preauthorization: the submission of a dental insurance claim requesting permission and/or allowed monies designated for specific procedures prior to the actual delivery of the procedure.

Preceptorship: entails training on the job, by an employer, then receiving licensure after passing a written test.

Preferred provider organization: an organization where a dentist or provider agrees to provide dental care to patients enrolled in the plan at discounted fees. In return the dentist or provider is given access to a pool of patients who have the dental coverage.

Prima facie: at first sight; moral obligation that appears from first sight as compelling but may be overridden by stronger duties.

Privilege: valid claim earned by effort and hard work.

Production: the total amount or costs of services given to patients. Production can be calculated by the day, week, month, or year.

Professional negligence: malpractice; not performing standard of care and harm results; part of tort law, civil law.

Public relations: the promotion and protection of a company's image.

Resume: a summary of facts: education, employment, memberships, qualifications

Rights: valid claims guaranteed in a society.

Risk management: term used to describe the actions taken to prevent financial loss or possible legal action.

Rule utilitarian: a utilitarian who is concerned with the rule from which an action is derived.

Slander: verbal (oral, spoken) defamation; one of two types of defamation, the other being libel (written).

Spouse abuse: domestic violence; battered wife; control over an intimate individual.

Standard negligence: ordinary negligence; negligence that does not involve patient care or professional responsibilities.

State assistance: A state funded program for qualified consumers that will allow health and dental care delivery at no cost to the consumer.

Statutory law: law enacted by legislation; two types of statutory law are criminal law and civil law.

Surrogate: legal representative for patient (i.e., minor or incompetent individual).

Team concept: the idea that all members act as part of a team and work to attain a common goal.

Technical assault: touching without permission, but with no intention of harming; similar to technical battery.

Technical battery: touching without permission, but with no intention of harming; similar to technical assault.

Teleology: consequentialism; branch of normative ethics that emphasizes consequences of an action.

Tort: civil wrong; can be intentional or unintentional; part of civil law.

Trust: confidence in the truth or action; a core value or ethical principle found in a code of ethics.

Usual, reasonable and customary: refers to the fees a dentist will charge for the services offered to consumers.

Utility: usefulness of an action; underlies the theory of utilitarianism.

Veracity: telling the truth; a core value or ethical principle found in a code of ethics.

Virtue ethics: type of ethics that places emphasis on character traits of the person rather that the behavior.

Works Cited

American Dental Hygienists' Association. Division of Governmental Affairs. Stateline. (1996). *Access, 10*(10), 38–39.

American Dental Association. (1998). *Proceedings: Dentists C.A.R.E. Conference.* Chicago: Author.

American Dental Hygienists' Association. (1999). *Bylaws and code of ethics.* Chicago: Author.

Ashur, M. S. (1993). Community oriented primary care approach to domestic violence. *Journal of the American Medical Association, 296*(18), 2367.

Babinski, D. (1999). Bridge Network, Inc. Dental Products and Services. *http://www.bridge-network.com.*

Bebeau, M. J., Rest, J. R., & Yamoor, C. M. (1985). Measuring dental students' ethical sensitivity. *Journal of Dental Education, 49*(4), 225–235.

Bergmann, T. (2000). The beauty of managed care. *RDH,* 20(6), 46–45, 100.

Bressman, J. K. (1993). Risk management for the '90s. *Journal of the American Dental Association, 124*(3), 63–67.

Centers for Disease Control. (1990). Recommendations for preventing transmission of human immunodeficiency virus and hepatitis B virus to patients during exposure-prone invasive procedures. *Morbidity and Mortality Weekly Report, 40*(No. RR-8, July 12), 1–9.

Centers for Disease Control. (1998). Are patients in a dentist's or doctor's office at risk of getting HIV? *http://www.cdc.gov/hiv/pubs/faq/faq29.htm.* Retrieved October 1, 2001.

Commission on Dental Accreditation (1998). *Accreditation Standards for Dental Hygiene Programs.* Chicago: American Dental Association.

Covey, S. (1990). *The 7 habits of highly effective people: Restoring the character ethic.* New York: Simon & Schuster.

Curley, A. W. (1997). Malpractice: The dentist's perspective. *Journal of the American College of Dentists, 64*(2), 21–24.

Curran, A. E., & Darby, M. (1990). Dental hygiene preceptorship: An issue of risk management. *Journal of Dental Hygiene, 64*(7), 290–295.

da Fonseca, M. A., & Idelberg, J. (1993). The important role of dental hygienists in the identification of child maltreatment. *Journal of Dental Hygiene, 67*(3), 135–139.

Darby, M. L. (Ed.). (1998). *Comprehensive review of dental hygiene* (4th ed.). St. Louis: Mosby.

Darby, M., & Walsh, M. (1995). *Dental hygiene theory and practice.* Philadelphia: Saunders.

Davison, J. A. (2000). *Legal and ethical considerations for dental hygienists and assistants.* St. Louis: Mosby.

Dean Witter. (2000). General investment information. *http://www.deanwitter.com. Dental Products Report.* (1999, July).

DesAutels, P., Battin, M., & May, L. (1999). *Praying for a cure: When medical and religious practices conflict.* Lanham, MD: Rowman & Littlefield.

DeVore, C. (1997). Legal risk management for the dental hygienist. *The Journal of Practical Hygiene 6*(4), 59–61.

Dietz, E. (2000). *Dental office management.* Albany, NY: Delmar Publishers.

Edelman, M. A., & Menz, B. L. (1996). Selected comparisons and implications of a national rural and urban survey in health care access, demographics, and policy issues. *Journal of Rural Health, 12*(3), 197–205.

Elderly Abuse & Neglect Program. (1991). *Elderly Abuse Awareness.* Springfield: The Illinois Department on Aging.

Emmot, L. (1999). Boys & toys. *RDH* (Oct.), 81–86.

Ganssle, C. L. (1995). *Managing oral healthcare delivery: A resource for dental professionals.* Albany, NY: Delmar Publishers.

Garvin, C., & Siedge, S. H. (1992). Sexual harassment within dental offices in Washington state. *Journal of Dental Hygiene, 66*(4), 178–184.

Gatson, M. A., Brown, D. M., and Waring, M. B. (1990). Survey of ethical issues in dental hygiene. *Journal of Dental Hygiene, 64*(5), 217–224.

Gibson-Howell, J. C. (1996). Domestic violence identification and referral. *Journal of Dental Hygiene, 70*(2), 74–77.

Glantz, L., Mariner, W., & Annas, G. (1992). Risky business: Setting public health policy for HIV-infected health care professionals. *The Milbank Quarterly, 70*(1), 43–79.

Gutheil, T., & Appelbaum, P. (1998). Confidentiality and privilege. In *Clinical handbook of psychiatry and the law.* New York: McGraw-Hill.

Hanks, P. (Ed.). (1986). *The Collins English dictionary* (2nd ed.). London: William Collins Sons & Co.

Haring, J. I., & Jansen, L. (2000). *Dental radiography: Principles and techniques* (2nd ed.). Philadelphia: Saunders.

Hazel, C. (1998). The vital role of practice marketing. Hycomb Marketing Tools for Dentists. *http://www.hycomb.com.*

Highlander Dental. (2000). Dental Equipment Sales and Service. Redding, California.

Honderich, T. (Ed.). (1995). *The Oxford companion to philosophy.* New York: Oxford University Press.

Illinois Department of Professional Regulation. (2000). *Rules for the administration of the Illinois Dental Practice Act.* Springfield: State of Illinois.

Illinois Department on Aging. (1999). *Elderly abuse . . . It happens.* Springfield: State of Illinois.

Johnson, O. N., McNally, M. A., & Essay, C. E. (1999). *Essentials of dental radiography for dental assistants and hygienists* (6th ed.). Stamford, CT: Appleton & Lange.

Kessler, H., Bick, J., Pottage, J., & Benson, C. (1992). AIDS: Part 1. *Disease-a-Month, 38*(9), 633–639.

Knapp, K. K., & Hardwick, K. (2000). The availability and distribution of dentists in rural zip codes and primary care health professional shortage areas (PC-HPSA) zip codes: Comparison with primary care providers. *Journal of Public Health Dentistry, 60*(1), 43–48.

Kohlberg, L. A. (1967). Moral and religious education and the public school: A developmental view. In T. Sizer (Ed.), *Religion and public education.* Boston: Houghton-Mifflin.

Kotler, P. (1997). *Marketing management: Analysis, planning, implementation and control* (9th ed.). Upper Saddle River, NJ: Prentice Hall.

LeBlanc, H. P., Nawrot, R., Bernstein, F., Mumford, S., Lautar, C., & Beaver, S. (1997). *Southern seven oral health needs assessment.* Unpublished study. Center for Rural Health and Social Services Development, Southern Illinois University, Carbondale, Illinois.

Litch, C. S., & Liggett, M. L. (1992). Consent for dental therapy in severely ill patients. *Journal of Dental Education, 56*(5), 298–311.

Loesche, W. L. (1997). Association of the oral flora with important medical diseases. *Current Opinion in Periodontology, 4, 21–28.*

Masek, R. T. (1999). Cutting time and expenses with the Cerec 2 CAD/CAM system. *Dentistry Today, 18*(4), 64–68.

McKee, L. (2000). Workplace issues. *Access, 14*(6), 16–24.

Miles, L. (1999). CEO practice management consultant. *http://lindamiles. worldnet.att.net.*

Miller, R. D., & Hutton, R. C. (2000). *Problems in health care law* (8th ed.). Gaithersburg, MD: Aspen Publishers.

Mueller-Joseph, L., & Peterson, M. (1995). *Dental hygiene process: Diagnosis and care planning.* Albany, NY: Delmar Publishers.

Munson, R. (1996). *Interventions and reflection: Basic issues in medical ethics* (5th ed.). Belmont, CA: Wadsworth.

Neiburger, E. J. (1998). How to profit from computers: 10 rules for selecting a computer system. *Dental Economics.* Pen Well. (Aug.), 96–99.

Nelson, D. M. (2000). *Review of dental hygiene.* Philadelphia: Saunders.

Newell, K. J., Young, L. J., & Yamoor, C. M. (1985). Moral reasoning in dental hygiene students. *Journal of Dental Education, 49*(2), 79–84.

Newman, J. F., & Gift, H. C. (1992). Regular pattern of preventive dental services—A measure of access. *Social Science and Medicine, 35*(8), 997–1001.

Nierenberg, J. (1999). Women and the art of negotiating. The Negotiation Institute. *http://www.negotiation.com.*

Ohio State Dental Board. (2000). *Ohio State Dental Board law and rules.* Columbus: State of Ohio.

Oldenquist, A. G. (1978). *Moral development: Text and readings* (2nd ed.). Boston: Houghton-Mifflin.

Ozar, D. T., & Sokol, D. J. (1994). *Dental ethics at chairside: Professional principles and practical applications.* St. Louis: Mosby.

Paige, B. E. (1977). Malpractice: An overview for the dental hygienist. *Dental Hygiene, 51*(4), 167–173.

Patients' Bill of Rights Act of 1999. U.S. Congress (July 8). Washington, DC: U.S. Government Printing Office.

Peck, S. B. (2000). Testimony before the House Appropriations subcommittee on labor, health and human services, education and related agencies on fiscal year 2001 appropriations. *Access, 14*(6), 41–43.

Pollack, B. R., & Marinelli, R. (1988). Ethical, moral and legal dilemmas in dentistry: The process of informed decision making. *Journal of Law and Ethics in Dentistry, 1*(1), 27–36.

Pollack, B. R., & Marinelli, R. D. (1988). Ethical, moral, and legal dilemmas in dentistry: The process of informed decision making. *Journal of Law and Ethics in Dentistry, 1*(1) 27–36.

Public Health Futures Illinois. (2000). *Illinois plan for public health systems change.* Springfield: Authority State of Illinois.

Purtilo, R. (1999). *Ethical dimensions in the health professions* (3rd ed.). Philadelphia: Saunders.

Rauls, J. (1971). *A theory of justice.* Cambridge, MA: The Belknap Press of Harvard University Press.

Raveal, M. (1989). Dental hygiene regulation and practice. *Journal of Public Health Dentistry, 49*(4), 228–230.

Reis-Schmidt, T. (1998). Trends in dentistry. *Dental Products Report* (Aug.), 24–31.

Rest, J. R. (1986). *Moral Development: Advances in research and theory.* New York: Praeger Publishers.

Rest, J., Narvaez, D., Bebeau, M., & Thoma, S. (1999). A neo-Kohlbergian approach: The DIT and schema theory. *Educational Psychology Review, 11*(4), 291–324.

Rich, J. M., & DeVitis, J. L. (1985). *Theories of moral development.* Springfield, IL: Charles C. Thomas.

Rosoff, A. (1981). *Informed consent: A guide for health care providers.* Rockville, MD: Aspen Systems Corp.

Rule, J. T., & Veatch, R. M. (1993). *Ethical questions in dentistry.* Chicago: Quintessence.

Saxe, M. D., & McCourt, J. W. (1991). Child abuse: A survey of ASDC members and a diagnostic-data-assessment for dentists. *Journal of Dentistry for Children, 58*(5), 361–366.

Schwimmer, A., Massoumi, M., & Barr, C. E. (1994). Efficacy of double gloving to prevent inner glove perforation during outpatient oral surgical procedures. *Journal of the American Dental Association, 125*(2), 196–198.

Scott, B. L. (1999). Ethics dialogue in dental hygiene. *Access, 13*(10), 14–22.

Scott, R. (1998). *Professional ethics: A guide for rehabilitation.* St. Louis: Mosby.

Scott, R. W. (2000). *Legal aspects of documenting patient care* (2nd ed.). Gaithersburg, MD: Aspen Publishers.

Seckman, C. H. (2000). Don't call them disabled; call them practicing hygienists! *RDH, 20*(1), 34–38, 78.

Switankowsky, I. (1998). *A new paradigm for informed consent.* Lanham, MD: University Press of America.

The Motley Fool. (1999). Investments. *http://www.netscape.com/investing.*

U.S. Department of Health and Human Services. (2000). *Oral health in America: A report of the Surgeon General—Executive summary.* Rockville, MD: U.S. Department of Health and Human Services, National Institute of Dental and Craniofacial Research, National Institutes of Health.

Wagner, L. (1995). Bringing high technology down to earth. *Access— American Dental Hygienists Association* (Apr.), 22–31.

Weinstein, B. D. (1993). *Dental Ethics.* Philadelphia: Lea & Febiger.

Wilkins, E. (1999). *Clinical practice of the dental hygienist* (8th ed.). Philadelphia: Lippincott Williams & Wilkins.

Other References

Ahronheim, J. C., Moreno, J. D., & Zuckerman, C. (2000). *Ethics in clinical practice* (2nd ed.). Gaithersburg, MD: Aspen Publishers.

Alty, C. (1997). Mirror, mirror, on the wall, what is the most secure of all? *RDH* (Mar.), 16–20.

Alty, C. (1999). Who we are. *RDH* (Oct.), 64–64.

American Academy of Dental Practice Administration. (1999). History of the Academy. *http://www.aadpa.org*.

Baab, D. A., & Ozar, D. T. (1994). Whistleblowing in dentistry: What are the ethical issues? *Journal of the American Dental Association, 125*(2), 199–205.

Baily, B. (1995). Informed consent in dentistry. *Journal of the American Dental Association, 110*(5), 709–713.

Bebeau, M. J., & Thoma, S. J. (1999). Intermediate concepts and the connection to moral education. *Educational Psychology Review, 11*(4), 343–360.

Bernhardt, C. (1997). Creating an effective hygiene department. Welmar, CA: Christine Bernhardt & Associates.

Brill, B. (2000). Dentistry—The past 25 years. *http://www.dentalxchange.com*.

Byers, M. (1993). I'm a dentist and I'm HIV-positive. *Illinois Dental Journal, 62*(2), 81–84.

Carter-Hanson, C. (2000). Community oral health. In D. M. Nelson, *Saunders review of dental hygiene* (pp. 542–578). Philadelphia: Saunders.

Chandler, R. C. (1999). Deontological dimensions of administrative ethics, revisited. *Public Personnel Management, 28*(4), 505–514.

Chiodo, G., & Tolle, S. (1992). Can a rational patient make an irrational choice? The dental amalgam controversy. *General Dentistry, 40*(3), 184–187.

Chiodo, G., & Tolle, S. (1992). Diminished autonomy: Can a person with dementia consent to dental treatment? *General Dentistry, 40*(5), 372–373.

Ciesielski, C., Gooch, B., Hammett, T., & Metler, R. (1991). Dentist, allied professionals with AIDS. *Journal of the American Dental Association, 122*(9), 42–44.

Clark, K. (1999). Gimme, gimme, gimme. U.S. News Online. *http://www. usnews.com.*

Colby, A., & Kohlberg, L. (1987). *The measurement of moral judgment* (Vols. I & II). New York: Cambridge University Press.

Cortes, M. (1999). Nd:Yag laser-assisted gingivectomy, bleaching, and porcelain laminates, Part 2. *Dentistry Today 18*(4), 52–55.

Dalton, R. Public relations. American Laser Technologies.

Daniels, N. (1992). HIV-infected health care professional: Public threat, public sacrifice. *The Milbank Quarterly, 70*(1), 3–42.

Dental Practice & Finance. (1996, Nov./Dec.), 59.

Dentrix. (2000). Software systems for dental practice management. *http:// www.dentrix.com.*

Drevenstedt, M. S. (1999). When broken appointments shatter profitability. *Practice Management* (Mar./Apr.), 46–50.

Eaglesoft. (2000). Software systems for dental practice management. *http://www.eaglesoft.com.*

Eastman, S. (1999). Program director, Taft college Dental Hygiene, Taft, California. Interview.

Farmer, T. (1998). Getting paid what you're worth. *Access—American Dental Hygienists' Association* (June), 25–30.

Farr, C. (2000). Steps to creating the perfect high-tech practice, Part I. *http://www.dentalxchange.*

Finkbeiner, B. L., & Finkbeiner, C. A. (1996). *Practice management for the dental team* (4th ed.). St. Louis: Mosby.

Fredekind, R., Cuny, E., Peltier, B., & Carpenter, W. (1999). The hepatitis B antigen-positive dental school applicant. *Journal of Dental Education, 63*(10), 766–770.

Fudge, R. S., & Schlacter, J. L. (1999). Motivating employees to act ethically: An expectancy theory approach. *Journal of Business Ethics, 18*(3), 295–304.

Gairola, G. & Skaf, K. O. (1983). Ethical reasoning in dental hygiene. *Dental Hygiene, 57*(2), 16–20.

Gaston, M., Brown, D., & Waring, M. (1990). Survey of ethical issues in dental hygiene. *Journal of Dental Hygiene, 64*(3), 217–224.

Gellermann, W., Frankel, M. S., & Ladenson, R. F. (1990). *Values and ethics in organization and human systems development.* San Francisco: Jossey-Bass.

Gerbert, B., Bleecker, T., Miyasaki, C., & Maguire, B. (1991). *Journal of the American Medical Association, 265*(14), 1845–1848.

Gilligan, C. (1982). *In a different voice.* Cambridge, MA: Harvard University Press.

Goslin, D. A. (Ed.). (1969). *Handbook of socialization theory and research.* Chicago: Rand McNally.

Halsband, E. (1984). An introduction to problems of dental ethics. *Medicine and Law, 3*(4), 377–381.

Henry, P. (1992). Who speaks for the children?: Consent for treatment of minors. *Nurse Practitioner Forum, 3*(1), 4–5.

Hirsch, A., & Gert, B. (1986). Ethics in dental practice. *Journal of the American Dental Association, 113*(4), 599–603.

James, K. R. (1999). How can I find the right employees? *Journal of the American Dental Association,* Vol. 130, 1101–1103.

Jones-Emmerling, H. (1996). A job to die for. *RDH* (May), 22–26.

Jones, D. (1993). The whole truth or nothing? A tale of misinformed consent. *Journal of the Canadian Dental Association, 59*(7), 592–595.

Jones, L. (1999). Retirement planning: What do you want to do with the rest of your life? *http://www.WomenCONNECT.com.*

Jones, T. M. (1991). Ethical decision making by individuals in organizations. *The Academy of Management Review, 16*(2), 366–395.

Knapp, M. (1988). Decision making by and for nursing home residents. *Clinics in Geriatric Medicine, 4*(3), 667–679.

Kohlberg, L. A. (1958). *The development of modes of moral thinking and choice in the years 10–16.* Unpublished doctoral dissertation, University of Chicago.

Lacey, A. R. (1986). *A dictionary of philosophy* (2nd ed.). New York: Routledge.

Lautar, C. J., & Pimlott, J. F. L. (1998). Periodontal diagnosis and care planning. In K. O. Hodges (Ed.), *Concepts in nonsurgical periodontal therapy* (pp. 153–179). Albany, NY: Delmar Publishing.

Layman, E. (1996). Ethics education: Curricular considerations for the allied health discipline. *Journal of Allied Health, 25*(2), 149–160.

Logan, M. (1993). Infectious diseases: Answers to ten legal (or illegal?) questions. *Illinois Dental Journal, 62*(1), 19–21.

Milestone Scientific. (1997). The Wand: Computer controlled local anesthetic delivery system. Professional informational brochure.

Morganstein, W. (1976). Informed consent: The doctrine evolves. *Journal of the American Dental Association, 93*(3), 637–642.

Nash, D. (1984). Ethics in dentistry: Review and critique of principles of ethics and code of professional conduct. *Journal of the American Dental Association, 109*(4), 597–603.

Nathe, C., & Posler, B. (1999). A spirit of collaboration . . . and, yes, independence. *RDH* (July), 20.

Nelson, B. (2000). Evaluating the team member's role. *http://www.smartbiz.com.*

Nierenberg, J. (1999). Women and the art of negotiating. The Negotiation Institute. *http://www.negotiation.com.*

O'Connell, B. (1989). When patients refuse treatment. *Journal of Dental Hygiene, 63*(1), 38–39.

Odom, J. (1991). Ethics and dental amalgam removal. *Journal of the American Dental Association, 122*(7), 69–71.

Odom, J., Odom, S., & Jolly, D. (1992). Informed consent and the geriatric dental patient. *Special Care in Dentistry, 12*(5), 202–206.

Ostuni, W., & Mohl, G. (1995). Communicating more effectively with the confused or demented patient. *General Dentistry, 43*(3), 264–266.

Pence, G. (1995). *Classic cases in medical ethics* (2nd ed.). New York: McGraw Hill.

Pitchard, M. S. (1999). Kohlbergian contributions to educational programs for the moral development of professionals. *Educational Psychology Review, 11*(4), 395–409.

Price, D. (1991). What should we do about HIV-positive health professionals? *Archives of Internal Medicine, 151*(4), 658–659.

Rada, R., & Jankowski, B. (1993). Attitudes, practice and employer responsiveness toward infection control as seen by certified dental assistants in Illinois. *Illinois Dental Journal, 62*(2), 89–93.

Rest, J. R. (1979). *Development in judging moral issues.* Minneapolis: University of Minnesota Press.

Rest, J. R. (1982). Psychologist looks at the teaching of ethics. *The Hastings Center Report, 12*(1), 29–36.

Rest, J. R. (1983). Morality. In P. H. Mussen (Ed.), *Handbook of child psychology* (4th ed., Vol. 3, pp. 556–629). New York: Wiley.

Rest, J. R. (1990). *DIT manual* (3rd ed.). Minneapolis: Center for the Study of Ethical Development.

Rest, J. R. (1999). *Postconventional moral thinking: A neo-Kohlbergian approach.* Mahwah, NJ: Erlbaum.

Rest, J. R., & Narvaez, D. (Eds.). (1994). *Moral development in the professions: Psychology and applied ethics.* Hillsdale, NJ: Erlbaum.

Rest, J., Thoma, S., & Edwards, L. (1997). Designing and validating a measure of moral judgment: Stage preference and stage consistency approaches. *Journal of Educational Psychology, 89*(1), 5–28.

Robbins, S. P. (1998). *Organizational behavior* (8th ed.). Upper Saddle River, NJ: Prentice Hall.

Robin, B. (1998). *Personnel manual for the dental office employee.* Los Angeles: Author.

Rowe, M. (1997). Dental fear and HIV contagion. *Journal of Practical Dental Hygiene, 6*(5), 47–48.

Ryan, R. (2000). Background check. *http://www.WomenCONNECT.com.*

Ryan, R. (2000). Choose me! Don't let your resume be just another piece of paper in the pile. *http://www.WomenCONNECT.com.*

Schoeffel, A. (1998). Discrimination: Exposure-prone procedures and HIV-infected health care professionals. *American Journal of Law and Medicine, 24*(1), 127–129.

Schulman, D. (1991). HIV-infected health care providers: Legal rights and protections. *Annals of Emergency Medicine, 20*(12), 1379–1381.

Seckman, C. (1999). Bossy questions: The most important part of a job interview may well be the questions you ask. *RDH* (Nov.), 24–27.

Sfikas, P. (1996). Guarding the files: Your role in maintaining the confidentiality of patient records. *Journal of the American Dental Association, 127*(8), 1248–1252.

Shick Technologies, Inc. (2000). Digital radiology systems. *http://www.shicktech.com.*

Shuman, S. (1989). Ethics and the patient with dementia. *Journal of the American Dental Association, 119*(6), 747–748.

Shuman, S., & Bebeau, M. (1994). Ethical and legal issues in special patient care. *Dental Clinics of North America, 38*(3), 553–575.

Smith, T. J. (1988). Informed consent doctrine in dental practice: A current case review. *Journal of Law and Ethics in Dentistry, 1*(3), 159–169.

Starcevich, M., & Stowell, S. J. (1997). Boosting commitment in your team. *Entrepreneurial Edge* (3). *http://www.edge.lowe.org.*

Stevens, M. M. (1998). Massage helps relieve aching muscles, so why not invite a therapist to the office? *RDH* (June), 56–60.

Stevens, M. M. (1996). Harmony in hygiene. *RDH* (Dec.), 26–29.

Thoma, S. J., & Rest, J. R. (1999). The relationship between moral decision-making and patterns of consolidation and transition in moral judgment development. *Developmental Psychology, 35*(2), 323–334.

Veatch, R. (1985). The relationship of the profession to society. *Journal of Dental Education, 49*(4), 207–213.

Von Buol, P. (1999). Dental hygienists' business savvy boosts practice success. *Access—American Dental Hygienists Association* (Mar.), 26–30.

Wakeen, L. M. (1993). Dental office emergencies: Do you know your legal obligations? *Journal of the American Dental Association, 124*(8), 54–57.

Wear, S. (1998). *Informed consent: Patient autonomy and clinician beneficence within health care* (2nd ed.). Washington, DC: Georgetown University Press.

Westwick, G. M. (1999). Retired periodontist, Taft College Dental Hygiene, Taft, California. Interview.

Windsor, J. C., & Cappel, J. C. (1999). A comparative study of moral reasoning. *College Student Journal, 33*(2), 281–287.

Wolfe, F. D. (1999). Painful Inspiration. *RDH* (Nov.), 34–50.

Woodall, I. R. (1987). *Legal, ethical, and management aspects of the dental care system* (3rd ed.). St. Louis: Mosby.

Woodman, R., & Malz, V. (1994). Informed consent and the elderly dental patient. *Special Care in Dentistry, 14*(2), 65–67.

Yen, T-W. (1998) Faster than an x-ray, safer than . . . well, an x-ray. *Dental Economics.* Pen Well. (Aug.), 46–50.

Zarkowski, P., & Shepherd, K. R. (1990). Legal considerations and preceptorship: Not to be ignored. *Journal of Dental Hygiene, 64*(10), 358–364.

Index

attire, 180–81
employer considerations, 176
expectations, outlining prior to
   interview, 178
legal aspects, 176–77
listening carefully, 177
personality tests, 180
positive attitude, importance of,
   177
questions, preparing pertinent,
   178–79
techniques, 174–76
working interviews, advantages,
   179–80
Intraoral cameras
components, 155
cost, 155
disadvantages, 157–58
mobile versus stationary systems,
   155
patient education, 156–57
Tips for operation, 158
uses, in the dental practice, 157
Investment planning
compounding interest, 199
initial steps, 198–99
investment brokers, 201
investment vehicles, 200–201
online trading, 201
pitfalls, 202
risk factors, 199, 201

J

Jurisprudence, 68
Justice
and access to care, 101–3
compensatory, 103
as a core value, 25
distributive, 102
procedure, 103
social (Rawls), 12–16
utilitarian view, 9

K

Kant, Immanuel (1724–1804), 6–7
Kantian ethics. *See also* Deontology

and autonomy, 20
categorical imperatives, 7
consequences, irrelevancy to moral
   values, 6
moral duties, 6–7
Kohlberg's model of moral development, 57–59
cognitive development, 58–59
levels and stages, 57–58

L

Libel, 74
Licensure
certification, 81
credentialing, 80–81
educational requirements, 78–79
practical board examinations,
   79–80. *See also* Appendix B:
   217–18; Appendix C: 219–220
reciprocity restrictions, 80
written board examinations, 79
Locke, John (1632–1704), 9–10

M

Malpractice
avoiding, 73
causes, 72
defined, 72
insurance, importance of, 73
proving, conditions necessary, 72
Managed care
capitation, 104, 142
defined, 104
DHMOs, 105, 142
plans, types of, 104
PPOs, 105, 141–42
Management styles
authoritative management, 115
Free-rein management, 116
participatory management, 116
Marketing. *See also* Profit centers
addressing questions of the consumer, 125
advertising, 126
defined, 124
education, importance of, 125